Dr. Deepak Dugar uncovers the truth that your beauty perceptions are shaped by advertising, social media, and the perceptions of people around us, and empowers you to filter those toxic inputs with a grateful mindset so you can accept and love yourself as you truly are: a beautiful human.

—Tony Robbins,

New York Times #1 Bestselling author of Unshakeable

Dr. Dugar is the rare human being (let alone plastic surgeon) who makes everyone around him feel beautiful with his kindness, empathy, and wisdom. Known for his immense skill in rhinoplasty, Dr. Dugar is actually a humanist who understands that the physical body is only one part of you, and he finds real meaning in making people feel good about their whole self. In his thought-provoking book, Dr. Dugar explores how culture, social media, and celebrities distort our self-images, and how confidence, humor, and perspective can give people their positive self-image back, often without surgery.

—Jeff Toll MD,

Celebrity Primary Care and Concierge Medicine Physician

I've always admired Dr. Deepak Dugar for his integrity and honesty, and those attributes shine brightly throughout his book, Be-YOU-tiful. I found it fascinating that Dr. Dugar turns more people away from surgery than those he actually operates on! What a fresh perspective from a celebrity Beverly Hills plastic surgeon! This book leaves a lasting impression, one that empowers readers to appreciate their beautiful uniqueness, not society's warped view of how they are supposed to look.

—Leslie Marcus,

Supervising Investigative Producer, The Doctors TV Show

It takes courage for a celebrity plastic surgeon from Beverly Hills to say, "You don't need surgery." But that's what Dr. Deepak Dugar does in Be-YOU-tiful: Flip the Script and Celebrate Your True Beauty. We've all carried the false narrative in our minds about the definition of true beauty and how we don't measure up. Dr. Dugar has written an empowering message to free us from those outside voices and to quiet those inner voices. He helps us to flip the script and begin to appreciate our own real beauty. He assures us that even on our worst days, we indeed are Be-YOU-tiful!

—Stephanie Mahin, Ph.D.,

Public Relations Specialist

The tricky thing about beauty is that it should be our right to choose how and what we do to our bodies. But, the scary thing is, we often don't know how influenced our beauty choices really are. We're living in a world of beauty peer pressure and pretending it's our idea that we need a surgery, an injection or something to make ourselves more beautiful...and I include myself in that category.

—Mia Khalifa,

Model, Actress, Sports Commentator, Social Media Influencer

Dr. Dugar always reminds me how beautiful I am, advocating to NOT get surgery—not a typical plastic surgeon. I'm so glad this book gets to show the world his love for his patients and the importance of self-love. He is always helping bring out the best you while reinforcing your confidence!

—LouLou Gonzalez,

Comedian, Actress, Writer

Be-YOU-tiful is an engaging and data-driven book packed with enlightening insights! It will challenge your perceptions of beauty by highlighting the ugly truth about the cosmetics, fashion, and diet industries and their harmful marketing practices. It will inspire you to love yourself and appreciate a natural approach to holistic beauty. As a professional in aesthetics, I respect and admire that Dr. Deepak Dugar can put his clients and their best interests ahead of his own. It's a wonderful read, and I highly recommend it!

—Tulsi Shah Bhargava, MSN, RN, AGNP

When a highly sought-after Beverly Hills plastic surgeon uses frank and honest conversation more than he uses his scalpel to help patients see their true beauty, it's worth taking notice! With compelling data and colorful stories, Dr. Dugar takes us behind the curtain to expose how culture, advertising, media, and even the people we choose to spend our time with influence us about what is beautiful.

—Shelby Howard, BSN,
Registered Aesthetic Nurse Injector

It is strange how being Dr. Dugar's patient, I feel the prettiest with my surgical nose and also the prettiest looking back at the photos before my surgery. He is not just a doctor to me, but a therapist in ways that are unimaginable. Is there really a difference between someone telling you "you don't look pretty" and going to a plastic surgeon and hearing all the things that they can do to improve your attractiveness? Imagine going to a celebrity plastic surgeon who has an encyclopedia of experiences, hearing him say every little thing that makes you beautiful and rejecting you for surgery because the expert himself believes in your beauty. Be-YOU-tiful feels like I am in a deep conversation with Dr. Dugar himself, unlocking every reason why I am so compelled to follow beauty standards to be considered "beautiful.

—Ishika Jain,

Former Patient, Mumbai, India

I wish I had read Deepak Dugar's Be-YOU-tiful earlier! I even wish I could go back in time with this book and read it to my younger self!!! I spent almost 12 years modeling in the fashion industry and never did a day go by without other people's judgments and perceptions of me, whether about how to change my face or why my body wasn't perfect. It led to years of looking at myself with a skewed perception of what beauty really meant. I look back on old photos of myself and wish I wasn't so hard on that girl trying to be what everyone was telling her she had to be in order to "make it" because she WAS and still IS beautiful. I am grateful for Deepak's powerful words and insight, his captivating, enlightening, and empowering perspective on beauty, and the opportunity to be able to accept his insight and use it while appreciating who I am and seeing how far I've come in my self-acceptance. I will be passing this knowledge on to my children in hopes of creating a world that reflects their beauty rather than society's morbid rendition. Deepak just gets it, and I couldn't be more grateful for the way in which Be-YOU-tiful has changed my self-image for the better.

—Nina Marie Danielle,
Actress, Comedian, Social Media Influencer

Be-YOU-tiful is an insightful and positive approach to helping individuals really understand that beauty is defined by self-confidence and focusing on your own inner worth. As a psychologist, it is nice to know that Dr. Dugar consults with potential patients focusing on positive features versus pushing for cosmetic procedures. His goal is to assess the reason for a change in appearance, and sometimes the end result is not pursuing cosmetic surgery, but rather addressing body image issues through mental health support.

—Reena B. Patel,

Parenting Expert, Psychologist & Author

What Deepak Dugar reveals in this enlightening and shocking book can absolutely transform your self-image. No matter your gender, age, or culture, this book is empowering and makes you aware of unrealistic beauty standards and how they can affect you. It's a powerful message that all of us should hear!

—Kenta Seki,

Celebrity Fitness Trainer

BEYOUTIFUL

FLIP THE SCRIPT AND
CELEBRATE YOUR TRUE BEAUTY

DEEPAK DUGAR, MD

BEVERLY HILLS CELEBRITY PLASTIC SURGEON

PRESS

In dedication to my amazing
patients and their vulnerability
which has taught me the truth
that feeling beautiful is far
greater than looking beautiful.

Contents

How Ugly Are You?

She was born with a mole above the corner of her left lip. From the time she became self-aware at all, it bothered her. Her sisters told her that it was an "ugly mark" because beauty marks can only be on the right side of the face.

On her first day of high school, a group of senior football players made fun of her, laughing that she had chocolate on her face. Many times during her childhood she asked her mom if she could have it removed, but always got the same reply: *You know what your mole looks like. You don't know what a scar will look like.*[1]

When she was a junior in high school, she got a job working at a local clothing store as a brand ambassador, a role that required a fashion show and photo shoot for the local newspaper. As a result of the exposure, another local photographer asked to take her photo for a university newspaper. He introduced her to a stylist to do her hair and makeup for the shoot. That stylist encouraged her to attend a beauty show where hairdressers cut and styled models' hair on stage. She signed up, thinking it would be fun.

The hairdresser that day ended up being a successful New York hairdresser. After giving her some pretty waves and good advice, he gave her her two agent names to contact. The first modeling agent had nice things to say and booked her for a test shoot; however, she suggested she have the mole removed. That only amplified her insecurity about it. She went ahead with the test shoot with the mole intact.

The hairdresser from that shoot showed some of her Polaroids to Marie Anderson, an agent at what eventually became Elite Model Management in Chicago. Marie saw potential and requested a meeting. When they met, Marie never said a word about the mole. The meeting resulted in one professional photo shoot, then another, and another—the jobs kept coming. A few times the mole was airbrushed out of printed photos. One time a makeup artist tried to cover it—only to have it look like a giant pimple. But as the modeling jobs increased, the mole simply stopped being mentioned at all.

Eventually, she appeared on the cover of the American *Vogue* magazine. At that point, she decided that if she looked good enough, mole and all, for the cover of arguably the most relevant fashion magazine, then she was good enough for everyone else. Some years later, as she reflected on her struggle with feeling insecure about her appearance, supermodel Cindy Crawford said, **"Isn't it ironic that the very thing that made me most insecure turned out to be my trademark?"**[2]

Cindy went on to be featured on a record-setting eighteen *Vogue* covers and countless others. This girl who grew up insecure about her looks nearly let the perspectives of other people define whether or not she was beautiful.

United by Ugly

It's hard to believe that at one point in her life, Cindy Crawford, a supermodel who was the face of "beautiful" for decades up to and into the new century, thought she was ugly. **But the ugly truth is this: every single person on this planet—supermodels included!—has at one time or another felt ugly.** I get it, *ugly* feels like a strong word, but it's the harsh word we often use when talking about ourselves to ourselves. Even if we don't say it out loud, deep down we may think it.

Have you ever looked in the mirror and seen something you didn't like? It's okay to admit it. You're not alone. Crow's feet. Nose bump. Freckles. Rosacea. Pimples. Grey hair. Thinning hair. Turkey neck. Droopy eyelids. Forehead lines. Thin lips. Big ears. High forehead. And that's just looking at the face!

Age spots. Breasts too big (or too small). Belly pooch. Fat rolls. Moles. Cellulite. Knock knees. Weird toes. Cankles. If I haven't already mentioned something you've criticized about yourself, I'd be surprised— and there are probably a few other things I didn't mention that also bug you about how you look.

Across the world, regardless of culture, age, race, gender, or any other category we use to divide ourselves, human beings are uniquely united in this one way: we have all felt less than beautiful at one time or another. The question is, *Why*?

As a plastic surgeon specializing in scarless rhinoplasty in Beverly Hills, California, I've had the privilege and opportunity to help a lot of people change their lives through surgery. But don't worry, this book is not about the merits of plastic surgery. We live in a culture where plastic surgery has become common because so many people are doing it. However, some of the most rewarding work I do is having frank conversations with people about just how beautiful they already are and explaining why they do not need surgery to make them beautiful. I know talking people out of surgery is, unfortunately, not a common practice for a plastic surgeon, but it is often the right thing to do.

Throughout my many years of practice, **I've interviewed over ten thousand people from all over the world and all different walks of life.** They meet with me because they think they want to surgically alter something about their appearances and are willing to accept the risks inherent in doing so. As people share their greatest insecurities with me about their physical appearances, our conversations often get deeply personal and usually reveal a deeper story.

One woman hates her nose because it looks just like the nose of her father who abused her when she was young. Another was bullied at school every day because of the bump on her nose and thinks if she can make the bump go away, all the hurtful memories will go with it. For some people, it's just a matter of wanting to look like someone they admire. Every situation is unique. **Sometimes I can change their lives with my scalpel; but often I can change their lives with a conversation about beauty and confidence.**

The truth is there are a lot of ideas out there about what beauty is and what it is not, who is beautiful and who is not. Unfortunately, too many people, perhaps even you, have fallen into the trap of thinking the question is not, *How beautiful am I?* but *Am I beautiful?* Ironically, feeling less than beautiful tends to leave us feeling isolated and alone when, in fact, we're all united in wrestling with the

Ironically,
feeling less than
beautiful tends
to leave us
feeling isolated
and alone when,
in fact, we're
all united in
wrestling with
the feeling that
we may not be
as beautiful as
we wish at times

feeling that we may not be as beautiful as we wish at times. All of us, even supermodels, feel ugly at some point in our lives. In the pages to come, I'll share more stories from other celebrities, influencers, and people just like you and me who've all struggled with feeling beautiful in some way, because I want you to know you are not alone. **Fighting that feeling of ugly is a universal human challenge.**

Taught to Be Beautiful

Our concepts of *ugly* have been programmed into us by our cultures. Our perceptions of *beauty* have been unconsciously shaped by voices around us. We've all been trained to think we have to look a certain way to be considered beautiful or good-looking. This is all taught to us, often at a young age.

Depending on where we live, we're taught different things. When we compare Asian cultures to Middle Eastern cultures to South American cultures, we see their concepts of beauty are dramatically different, not because of natural programming, but because of the way they were *taught* about beauty. Likewise, if we go to an African jungle culture where tribal leaders expect the females to elongate their necks using stacked rings, they're not doing that for fun. They're doing that because they have been taught that is how to become the most beautiful woman in the tribe.

These varied concepts of beauty exist for a wide variety of reasons, but the bottom line is that they are simply made-up, completely fabricated by social constructs. When we understand that those constructs exist and see them with a heightened self-awareness, we become empowered when it comes to how we think about our own appearance. For example, as you read these words, why are you wearing the clothing you have on right now? Why have you styled your hair the way you did today? Are you wearing make-up, or did you engage in some sort of personal grooming? Why? I suggest that those choices you made today about your appearance have been shaped by the social constructs that taught you to look a certain way.

Each of us has been shaped by these constructs. **It is this struggle to look and feel beautiful that unites us, but we must see the voices that shape us for what they are so we can**

free ourselves to be beautiful just as we are. Unfortunately, when it comes to assessing our own beauty, we tend to blindly follow the perceptions of others. For example, a young, twenty-something female once came to me for a consultation. She showed me pictures of people she follows on Instagram. She was obsessed with the shapes of their noses and wanted hers to look like theirs. But all the pictures she showed me were of girls who were pretty but had no relevance to the way this patient looks or should look.

Her example spotlights a problem we'll revisit later. Social media can be a dangerous place for beauty perception if you overexpose yourself to concepts of beauty that are probably filtered and not necessarily a natural fit for your personal genetic makeup. Depending on who you follow, you can create a social media landscape that is more inclusive to yourself, or you can make yourself feel more isolated and alienated.

Your closest real-life friends probably have similar interests and look a lot like you. You enjoy hanging out with them and feel like you "belong" when you are with them. You feel comfortable with them and experience positive energy from your encounters.

Contrast that with how you feel if you follow only the "beautiful" celebrities on social media with whom you have virtually nothing in common. You see them only after they've been worked over by their glam squad, perfectly positioned on their yacht, or flying around in a private jet—so you're not going to feel like you measure up. It can easily leave you feeling a little inferior, even ugly, when you compare yourself to someone else's perception of what it means to be beautiful.

But the reality is this: **Ugly is only a perception.** You are not ugly unless you think so. So, how ugly are you? That is entirely up to you.

Perhaps a better question is this: How beautiful do you want to be? Because the truth is, you already are.

It can easily
leave you
feeling a little
inferior, even
ugly, when
you compare
yourself to
someone else's
perception of
what it means
to be beautiful.

"What Bothers You?"

I realize it may seem odd to hear a plastic surgeon from Beverly Hills telling people they don't need surgery to be beautiful. But a lot of what I believe about telling the truth about beauty was shaped by my own story.

My dad grew up in a village in Rajasthan, India that had no electricity. One of eleven siblings, getting an education and a good job was the only way to escape poverty. He studied hard and became a "gold medalist", the equivalent to being a class valedictorian in America, but even more difficult to achieve. After he came to America and earned his engineering graduate degree, he returned to India to marry the woman who would become my mom. They returned to America and started a new life together.

I was the youngest of three kids. On the day I was born, my dad held me in his hands and said, "My third doctor!" (He was right. All three of us are doctors today.) I grew up in a small town called Beaumont in southeast Texas with a pretty "normal" upbringing. As an Eagle Scout, I loved spending a lot of time outdoors. I loved doing things with my hands and helping people.

My parents shaped who I became, each in their own unique way. From my dad, I learned the critical role of discipline and duty to success. My mom taught me to dream, think big, and change the world. She never cared about how much money we kids would make, what kind of car we'd drive, or what kind of house we'd live in. She only cared about each of her kids *being a good person.* I cannot tell you how many times I've heard those four words: **Be a good person. It seems so simple and such obvious advice, but it's another thing to live it, breathe it, talk it, and walk it.** Together they instilled a deep, deep sense of ethics into me that drives why I do or don't do certain things—including choosing not to operate on many patients.

As a teenager, I did have a defining experience that profoundly shaped how I saw the world around me. While our friends were vacationing in Europe or away at summer camp, my sister and I spent two consecutive summers at Mother Teresa's Missionaries of Charity orphanage in Calcutta, India. Every single day, we would sit with, take care of, and talk to kids living in poverty. Their parents or guardians had abandoned them at some point because they didn't have the ability, financially and or mentally, to care for them.

Working at Mother Teresa's orphanage was a trans-
formational experience in that it made me realize
both how fortunate I was and how much potential I
had to help people simply by talking with them. My
time there put things into perspective—suddenly not
getting invited to a classmate's birthday party wasn't
such a big deal when I saw children abandoned and
left in an orphanage.

From an early age, I sensed a desire to help people
by doing something meaningful with my hands that
would affect someone's life in a positive way. That's
why I made the choice after high school to pursue
plastic surgery. I went to a seven-year combined
medical program at George Washington University
in Washington, D.C. I did my surgical residency
training at the University of North Carolina at
Chapel Hill, a top-ten program in the country.

Then I did my fellowship for closed rhinoplasty
under Dr. Raj Kanodia, known as the celebrity guru
of rhinoplasty in Beverly Hills for the past forty years.
After I did my training under him, I started my own
practice in Beverly Hills. More than twelve years of
surgery and ten thousand patient interviews later, I
have done thousands of surgeries—not only in my

specialty of rhinoplasty, but also in other plastic surgeries. My practice has led me to work closely and confidentially with many celebrity names you would recognize, to be consulted as an expert by *E! News* and *The Doctors*, a syndicated television show, and to be featured in *Allure*, *The Huffington Post*, and more than forty-five other publications.

I say all that not to brag or impress, but simply to share that **beauty is my life's focus**. I'm not just a guy with an opinion about how people, women and men alike, should think about beauty. It's what I do all day, every day. As you'll see in the pages to come, I've engaged with thousands of people on this topic since my fellowship with my mentor, Dr. Raj Kanodia. Not only did he teach me everything I know about plastic surgery, but he also helped me understand the concept of beauty in terms of ethics and honesty because of how he practices. The first thing he helped me see was that as a plastic surgeon, it doesn't have to be only about surgery. It can really be about the conversation.

He would regularly say *no* to operating, telling people with such confidence how beautiful they are and that they didn't need surgery. When patients walked into the room, no matter what they looked like, he focused on their beautiful features. His approach contrasted with that of many plastic surgeons, who start a consultation by picking apart the patient to create the felt need for more surgery. What Dr. Kanodia would do—and what he taught me to do—was to immediately pick out all of someone's best features and share that with them. *I love your eyes. I love the way your lips look. I love your beautiful smile. Now, tell me what bothers you.*

And that's the second critical thing he taught me: never ever impregnate your perceptions of beauty into someone else's mind. Let them come to you with their perceptions. Let them bring it up. Many times people will come to see me and ask, *Just tell me, what do you think I should do?* I believe I have an ethical responsibility not to abuse my position and to evaluate who the person is and why they have come to me. If I sense someone is insecure and asking, *What would you do to me?,* my answer is always the same: *I wouldn't do anything. What bothers you?* That is the real question.

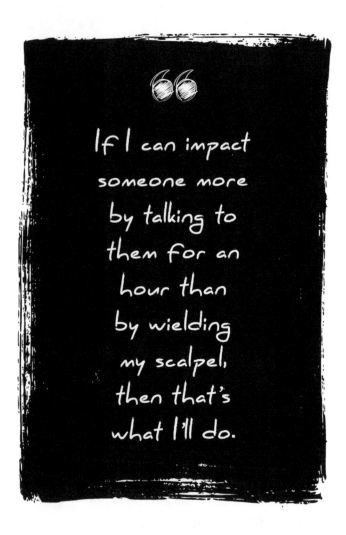

> If I can impact someone more by talking to them for an hour than by wielding my scalpel, then that's what I'll do.

As a plastic surgeon, people come to me at their most vulnerable. I can use that position for the good of the patient or for my own personal gain.

With my mom's voice in my head, and supported by Dr. Kanodia's example, I have always tried to wield my scalpel very carefully. I don't just pull it out because someone comes to me with insecurities they want fixed. A scalpel won't do that. I don't look at the money I could make, but at the *impact* I can make. If I can impact someone more by talking to them for an hour than by wielding my scalpel, then that's what I'll do.

It's not uncommon for people to fly from all over the world to see me. This past week alone I had three patients from London, one from Lima, Peru, and two from Dubai. They literally flew across the world to meet with me for surgery. When they arrived, I spoke bluntly and authentically with each of them as I always do. Regardless of the distance traveled, the consultation could result in my helping them realize they don't need the work done after all—and that revelation alone can be life-changing.

Beautiful Is Up to You

If there is one thing I have learned from studying beauty and people it is this: sometimes you need permission simply to be you. Instead of focusing on what you look like, how people perceive you, or how beautiful they think you are, you can actually become more aware of those voices that shape your perceptions of your beauty. Once you become aware of them, you can filter them and finally begin to relax instead of feeling like you have to conform to the expectations of others to be beautiful.

When you realize that we all struggle with some sort of insecurity about our physical appearance, from supermodels to teenagers to moms, dads, and grandparents, and that most of that insecurity comes from artificial expectations, you'll be equipped to finally break that frustrating cycle of trying to meet those shifting expectations.

No doubt you've heard it said, "Beauty is in the eye of the beholder." But what if beauty is actually in our own mind's eye? What if the only "beholder" that matters is you? Earlier I wrote that ugly is only a perception. Conversely, we could also say, beauty is only a perception. Everyone is beautiful who thinks they are. Just like it's up to you if you're ugly, it's up to you if you're beautiful.

In the pages to come, we'll explore what it means to be beautiful, both in Western culture and in cultures all around the world. We'll explore the voices that influence our perceptions of ugliness and beauty, both internal and external. I'll share with you the insights I share with patients who come from all over the world to consult with me. **Most importantly, I'll help you discover the truth that you are already beautiful and empower you to own it.** I want you to look in the mirror and acknowledge what is beautiful about the person looking back at you.

That doesn't mean it will be easy to break free from the prison of perceptions. But first, we need to see the ugly truth about beauty.

Beauty Notes

———

* Feeling less than beautiful tends
  to leave us feeling isolated
  and alone when, in fact, we're
  all united in wrestling with the
  feeling that we may not be as
  beautiful as we wish at times. All
  of us, even supermodels, feel
  ugly at some point in our lives.

* Our concepts of ugly have been
  programmed into us by our
  cultures. Our perceptions of beauty
  have been unconsciously shaped
  by voices around us. We've all been
  trained to think we have to look
  a certain way to be considered
  beautiful or good-looking.

✳ Sometimes you need permission
simply to be you. Instead of
focusing on what you look like,
how people perceive you, or
how beautiful they think you
are, you can actually become
more aware of those voices
that shape your perceptions of
your beauty. Once you become
aware of them, you can filter
them and finally begin to relax
instead of feeling like you have
to conform to the expectations
of others to be beautiful.

2

The Ugly Truth About Beauty

She traveled to Los Angeles from New York to meet me after five failed rhinoplasties; this consultation was for surgery number six. At this point, she seemed to simply be trying to find someone who could save her nose—but it went deeper than that. After just a few moments of speaking with her, I could tell that although everything in her world seemed to revolve around her nose, she really wanted someone to save *her*.

Her very first surgery happened when she was still a teen in the 1980s. Her Manhattan socialite mom had made her do it: "Your nose just isn't nice enough." For the next twenty-plus years of her life, she had a rhinoplasty about every three to five years. She would have the surgery, spend six months recovering, two years lamenting the results, and another year finding the next surgeon to visit. It was a vicious cycle in pursuit of what she thought would finally make her beautiful.

By the time I met her that day to discuss a sixth surgery, she was in her late forties or early fifties. I knew immediately I would not be doing surgery because it simply wasn't necessary. But we needed to have a deeper conversation. When I asked her what bothered her about her appearance, she offered a detailed analysis of her nose: *This nostril is higher than the other. The tip is asymmetric. This side dips in a little bit more right here with a little curve....* She went on and on, breaking down every single square millimeter of her entire nose.

Finally, I interrupted to deliver a little tough love: "Hold on! You're so hyper-focused on your nose right now, but you have to zoom out! Look at how beautiful your eyes are, and your cheeks, and your lips. Every part of your face is beautiful, and your nose fits. It works for your face. You've spent twenty years trying to make your nose something that it's not. Now after all these years and five surgeries, you still haven't achieved it. There is nothing you can do to your nose that will ever make it acceptable to you.

You just have to stop and accept that you are beautiful just the way you are."

Reading these words on this page can not fully convey the candid authenticity of my actual face-to-face conversation. But somehow, in that moment, I was able to help her see that it was time for her to just **stop** *chasing* **beauty and simply** *be* **beautiful**. She told me that of the more than thirty consults she'd had over her lifetime, I was the first surgeon who didn't simply agree with her that her nose needed work. She was looking for a perfect result, and frankly, that's like looking for a unicorn.

If someone comes to me who actually is a good candidate for a procedure, I let them know upfront that there is no such thing as a perfect result. *I'm very good at what I do and always do my best, but your anatomy will heal how it heals.* I never promise "the perfect nose" because that sets up unattainable expectations that can result in situations like the one I just described where someone tries endlessly to "get it right." I tell every patient before operating that surgery is generally one-and-done. There are no redos unless something bizarre happens, which is very rare. So, I set clear expectations early on.

You might be wondering how I decide who is and who isn't a good candidate for plastic surgery. Well, it really comes down to understanding a person's pain point and whether that pain point aligns with what is actually happening with their anatomy. For example, if a woman comes into my office with a tiny bump on her nose and yet says, *This is destroying my life! I can't live! I can't sleep! I can't eat or drink until it gets fixed!!* It's simply not going to happen. The significance of the anatomic issue does not match the level of this person's concern. There are often deeper emotional, mental, or psychological issues at work behind the perceptions that feel so real to them. I recommend that anyone seek professional help to evaluate those deeper concerns because there can be insecurity, self-confidence, or other issues going on beyond the perceived anatomical problem.

When perceptions are askew, we do not see ourselves as we truly are. Simply put, we have a shared problem of perception. If you have ever felt like you don't look beautiful enough, you are not alone. In fact, the ugly truth about beauty is that we are all united by the struggle to see ourselves as we truly are.

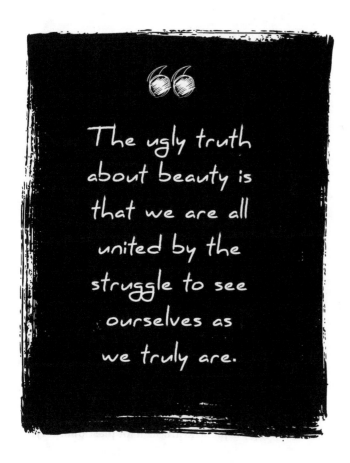

> The ugly truth about beauty is that we are all united by the struggle to see ourselves as we truly are.

An All-Consuming Pursuit

I hope that you have never had to experience cancer, either yourself or alongside a family member. If you have, you know it is all-encompassing. It dominates the patient's life and the lives of loved ones, too. All conversations seem to be about the patient's struggles and treatments. Given the life-or-death possibilities of a cancer diagnosis, that level of focus is understandable.

Unfortunately, it seems this chase for beauty can become like a mental cancer we bring upon ourselves. Many of the patients who have come to me experience their perceived flaws in the same all-consuming way, which, of course, is not mentally healthy. They feel compelled to check each flaw in the mirror dozens of times or more every day. They try to conceal it with makeup or clothing. They socially isolate themselves to keep the flaw (or their compulsive checking behavior) a secret. For 2 to 3% of the general population, this obsession devolves into a mental illness called Body Dysmorphic Disorder.[1] That percentage is more than double (7 to 8%) among people who are seen for plastic surgery.[2]

When someone comes to me who seems really focused in an unhealthy way on a beauty problem, I ask them to take a step back to check their perceptions. For example, when a patient is desiring a revision procedure on an already acceptable and harmonious anatomy, it carries a higher risk/benefit ratio, and I have to remind them: *Right now your nose* (or whatever it is) *bothers YOU - it doesn't bother anyone else. When you walk into a store or arrive at a party, nobody else notices it. They see a beautiful, wonderful person with an aura and energy ready to socialize. Or simply put, they just notice that you walked in. But if you continue down this path of revision surgery in pursuit of so-called perfection, and something goes wrong, or it ends up looking fake or botched, you'll walk through the door and EVERYONE will be bothered by your nose.*

It's all about perceptions. The reality is that if you think you look ugly, you are very likely the only person who shares your perception. And those who might agree with you do so because they have been influenced by the perceptions of others. There is a toxic self-deprecating culture that has permeated our society to feel *less* valued in our perceptions of ourselves instead of feeling *more* valued in our perceptions.

There is a toxic self-deprecating culture that has permeated our society to feel less valued in our perceptions of ourselves instead of feeling more valued in our perceptions.

Unfortunately, feeling ugly, or even less than beautiful, has far-reaching effects that go beyond feeling unhappy when we look in a mirror. Self-esteem expert Meaghan Ramsey revealed some truly staggering statistics from her research into body image in young girls:

> 60 percent of girls choose not to participate in activities because they think they don't look good enough; 31 percent withdraw from classroom debate so as not to draw attention to themselves if they believe they look bad; 20 percent skip class altogether when they feel unattractive, and research shows that girls who think they're fat get lower grades on tests than those who don't worry about this.[3]

Those numbers are staggering! **That means well over half of all girls change their life behavior significantly because they have a false perception of themselves.** Almost a third of them choose not to exercise their voices to avoid attention because they do not perceive themselves as being beautiful. And one in every five girls actually walks away from education opportunities because they perceive themselves as being less than attractive. These perceptions even affect their ability to think. That is both amazing and deeply disturbing!

From a young age, we are all conditioned by our environment and a number of voices (that we will unpack later) to pursue an ideal body image, encompassing everything from head to toe. That doesn't mean there actually is an ideal body or appearance, just perceptions and opinions on what is best. It is easy to generalize that younger adults would be the most confident in their appearance, as they tend to have the most coveted features. It would also be easy to assume college-educated people would have better control over their perceptions given the extent of their education. However, consider the following:

✱ Women are most likely to report being dissatisfied with how their bodies look (83% vs. 74% of men). *Did you get that?* **83% of women are dissatisfied with how their bodies look,** so if you are one of them, you are not alone.

✻ Younger adults are more likely to be dissatisfied with how their bodies look (86% of those ages 18-34 vs. 75% of those 55+)

✻ College graduates are more likely to be dissatisfied with how their bodies look (82% vs. 75% of those with no college degree).

✻ **Over 75% of adults would be willing to give up something they enjoy** or care deeply about to magically obtain their "perfect body."

✻ 85% of women and 79% of girls skip important activities due to body dissatisfaction.

✻ In South Africa, 64% of people feel comfortable in their own bodies. In the U.S., only 24% feel comfortable in their own bodies (ranked 9 out of 13 countries studied). **In Japan, a mere 8% feel comfortable in their own bodies.**[4, 5]

✻ Only 11% of girls around the world are comfortable describing themselves as beautiful. That number goes down as they age, to where **only 4% of women around the world actually consider themselves beautiful.**

✳ Ironically, 80% of women agree that every woman has something about her that is beautiful. Compare that with the numbers about self-perception above, and it is easy to see that women struggle to see their own beauty but can appreciate the beauty in others (more on this to come).

✳ More than half of women globally (54%) agree that when it comes to how they look, **they are their own worst beauty critic.**

Statistically speaking, body image issues are far more pervasive around the globe than any disease, including cancer. Does that surprise you? It seems that, as divided as the world often appears to be, there is something that unites us all—struggling with our perceptions of our own ugliness.

On one hand, that is shocking and sad; on the other hand, it may make you feel better knowing you are not the only one who struggles to see yourself as beautiful. **The good news is that when you learn to recognize the voices that shape your perceptions of yourself, you can filter them effectively and finally give yourself permission to enjoy being you.**

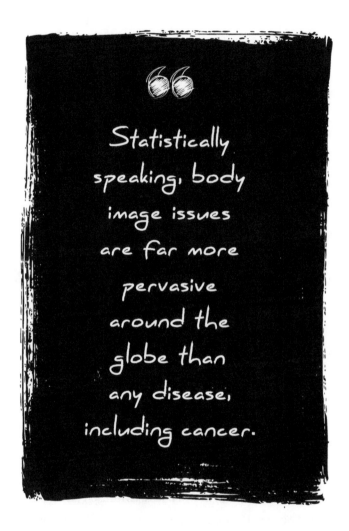

Statistically speaking, body image issues are far more pervasive around the globe than any disease, including cancer.

No one is immune from these distorted perceptions. For example, Jennifer Aniston, generally considered to be one of the most beautiful women in Hollywood—named *People Magazine*'s Most Beautiful Woman of the Year twice!—says, "I've never thought of myself that way [as being beautiful]. I didn't grow up being perceived that way, and I've certainly had many moments in my life where I didn't feel good enough or pretty enough or anything enough, where I felt horrible about myself."[6] Jennifer Lopez says, "It's hard to avoid comparing yourself to others, and I've definitely been guilty of it myself. I remember thinking I wasn't thin enough because I had curves."[7] Beyonce says, "After the birth of my first child, I believed in the things society said about how my body should look. I put pressure on myself to lose all the baby weight in three months, and scheduled a small tour to assure I would do it. Looking back, that was crazy."[8]

And it's not only women who struggle! Ryan Reynolds, dubbed one of *People Magazine*'s Sexiest Men Alive says, "I feel like an overweight, pimply-faced kid a lot of the time."[9] Likewise, Zac Efron says his first thought when he sees himself on screen is, "My head is huge."[10] Everyone shares in the struggle to want to feel beautiful yet fear they are only different shades of ugly.

Our perception
of beauty is
influenced by
a variety of
factors, including
evolutionary
preferences,
media influences,
cultural beliefs,
relationships
(community,
family, friends),
and individual
personality.

The Common Thread

A common thread unites the stories and statistics above and is at the heart of virtually every issue surrounding body image: *perception.* Our perception of beauty is influenced by a variety of factors, including evolutionary preferences, media influences, cultural beliefs, relationships (community, family, friends), and individual personality. To add to the confusion, **what is generally perceived as beautiful is always shifting,** and the toxicity of peer pressure to fit in waxes and wanes throughout life as well.

A 2017 study was conducted using functional MRI technology to see what happens in our brains when we perceive something or someone as beautiful.[11] Participants in the study were first asked to judge the luminance of a square to see if it was high or low. With that baseline established, they were then asked to judge a picture as either beautiful or ugly.

When participants looked at something they perceived to be beautiful, brain areas that govern perceptual, cognitive, emotional, and reward processing were activated. When looking at images they perceived to be ugly, only the visual areas of the brain were activated, demonstrating that the brain is selective and prefers to receive more stimulus from what it perceives to be beautiful.

An unanswered question from this study, however, is this: does our psychology activate these brain regions when we perceive beauty, or do our brain regions control the way we perceive beauty? It's an interesting question with no definite answer. **But one thing is clear: perceptions are literally central to how we think about beauty.**

Psychologist Aditya Shukla describes it this way:

> We are a product of evolution on Earth. Evolution promises us one thing: Variation. Variation in how we appear; how we think; how we behave. Everything about being ugly and beautiful lies in this fact. This variation allows us to have preferences, likes, and dislikes. Our brains are capable of making evaluations, attaching emotions to people, and passing judgment. These allow us to consider other people or objects as attractive or unattractive. In fact, it allows us to hold our own standards for beauty and ugliness... But, you are a product of evolution, and thus, you vary from others. It depends on you whether you want to call yourself ugly or beautiful. Judge only by your own standards, not someone else's. With that, you can choose to see yourself as ugly or pretty/beautiful.[12]

As you can see, the question of what is beautiful or what is ugly has no objective answer. Beauty is a relative concept. It depends on your perceptions. In the coming chapters, I will help you come to understand this more fully to free yourself from false standards of beauty so you will know the liberating truth:

You. Are. Beautiful. Right now. Just as you are.

And yes, I am talking to *you*.

Beauty Notes

* There is a toxic self-deprecating
  culture that has permeated
  our society to feel less valued
  in our perceptions of ourselves
  instead of feeling more
  valued in our perceptions.

* From a young age, we are all
  conditioned by our environment
  and a number of voices
  (that we will unpack later) to
  pursue an ideal body image,
  encompassing everything from
  head to toe. That doesn't mean
  there actually is an ideal body
  or appearance, just perceptions
  and opinions on what is best.

* Our perception of beauty is
  influenced by a variety of factors,
  including evolutionary preferences,
  media influences, cultural beliefs,
  relationships (community, family,
  friends), and individual personality.
  To add to the confusion, what is
  generally perceived as beautiful
  is always shifting, and the toxicity
  of peer pressure to fit in waxes
  and wanes throughout life as well.

* The good news is that when
  you learn to recognize the
  voices that shape your
  perceptions of yourself, you
  can filter them effectively
  and finally give yourself
  permission to enjoy being you.

3

Our Unifying Struggle

In a small tribal village in northern Namibia bordering Angola, Uvaserua awakens and begins her daily beauty ritual. She is a woman of the Himba, a tribe dubbed "the most beautiful tribe of Africa."[1] Uvaserua dresses in her sheepskin skirt and cowskin sandals. She remains topless.

She then begins applying Otjize paste, a cosmetic mixture of butterfat and ochre pigment to her entire body, including her hair plaits. Otjize is a highly desirable aesthetic beauty product, symbolizing the earth's rich red color and blood, the essence of life; it is the Himba ideal of beauty.[2] When she is thoroughly covered, she adds her traditional headpiece, necklaces, and beaded anklets. Feeling beautiful and ready for her day, she heads out to tend the cows and goats.

Meanwhile, in Seoul, South Korea, Sumin starts her day with a well-practiced skincare routine. She starts the ten-step process with a double cleansing, then exfoliates and applies toner, "essence", and serum. Next, she applies a sheet mask packed with beneficial vitamins and minerals. After removing the mask, she applies eye cream, moisturizer, and finally sunscreen.

After the entire routine is complete, Sumin slaps her face—the harder, the better—about fifty times to get the blood circulating and firm up her facial muscles. Finally, she reaches for her makeup: pearl-white iridescent eyeshadow to match her skin tone, doll-eye eyeliner, fruit-colored blush on the apples of the cheeks, and eyebrow pencil to achieve straighter eyebrows. Sumin uses three shades of lipstick to achieve a gradient with the darkest part in the center to enhance the natural appearance of her lips. Ready to face the day as her prettiest self, she heads out to school.

In another hemisphere, Ana is up early to head to the salon in Rio de Janeiro, Brazil, for her weekly visit. After stepping out of the shower and toweling off, she applies her Brazilian Bum Bum Cream for moisturizer. Noticing that her tan is fading, she makes a mental note that she needs to hit the beach this weekend. Giving her lips a quick swipe of Carmex, she heads out the door ready to go get made beautiful. She'll be getting her hair straightened, a manicure and pedicure, waxing, makeup (a natural look), and even lymphatic drainage (a way to avoid water retention achieved through sculpting massage).

Pick any city, town, or village in any country in the world, and you'll find a uniting principle: the pursuit of beauty. No matter the culture, all have a standard for beauty. You'll find the majority of women (and men, too!) taking steps each day to align with those unique cultural standards because there is no universal standard for beauty. Abby from San Francisco isn't going to feel beautiful covered head-to-toe in Otjize as Uvaserua does. You probably won't find Nubila from Islamabad slapping herself fifty times before she leaves home in the morning like Sumin. Priya from Mumbai isn't going to go lay on the beach for a tan as Ana does; instead, she's probably considering applying "Fair and Lovely" skin-lightening creams and avoiding the sun altogether to avoid getting "darker.".

All of these women are attempting to align with their cultural beauty standards, but where do these standards come from? And why do so many people feel ugly when they don't see themselves as measuring up? The answer to that question is neither simple nor straightforward.

Our Need for Validation

Over my many years of practice and more than ten thousand conversations with people about their perceptions of beauty, I have learned that **most perceptions and insecurities about how beautiful or ugly they are come from a need for external validation,** versus an internal validation and appreciation for who they are. External validation is related to why we want to look a certain way; internal validation is more about how we feel about ourselves when we look in the mirror. As a plastic surgeon, patients come to me for external validation, which requires me to be acutely aware of the influential position I am in and *never* misuse it.

One of my first professional mentors, Dr. Bruce Feldman, placed a significant emphasis on empathy.

He taught me that our first responsibility to our patients is to give them empathy; let them know they're not alone in what they are thinking and feeling. Give them that validation they are seeking. He saw every encounter as a human interaction more than a business interaction and taught me to never take that opportunity for granted.

In the last chapter, I shared the story of my patient who came to me for a consult looking for her sixth nose surgery, and I convinced her it wasn't necessary. You might be wondering how in a 20-minute conversation I could change the mind of someone who had spent years—decades, actually—believing she needed more surgery to be beautiful. It all comes down to *validation*.

I believe in that moment of our conversation she came to realize something she always knew deep down but never wanted to accept. It was almost as if she just needed to hear someone else—someone she viewed as an authority on the topic—say what she really believed but couldn't accept. **She was already beautiful.**

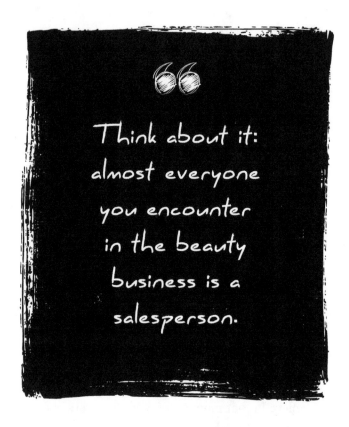

> Think about it: almost everyone you encounter in the beauty business is a salesperson.

The problem is that when you look into the external world for beauty validation, you're always being sold. As a result, rarely will someone talk to you honestly about beauty. Think about it: almost everyone you encounter in the beauty business is a salesperson. So, in this particular woman's case, when I spoke directly and honestly to her, it was as if she thought, *I've always kind of felt like that, but no one's ever said it to me.* After all, she had to understand that at some point, more surgery was absurd.

I think that encounter was the first time someone talked to her honestly from a professional standpoint. Perhaps she thought, *Wow, a plastic surgeon in Beverly Hills who makes money doing surgeries is telling me I'm OK!* I'm sure she was taken aback at first. The message of her beauty had never resonated externally because she had never heard it externally. She'd been depressed because of all the external sales and marketing telling her, *If you don't like it, just fix it.* I had the good fortune to be the right person at the right moment to provide healthy external validation.

Another potential patient came to consult with me. She was a young girl of 15. As I talked with her, I learned she was an average student who was a little less than motivated to succeed. She wasn't really popular and didn't have a lot of friends, so she was pretty down in the dumps. Her parents were clearly loving and concerned and had tried providing her with professional therapy since she was about eleven years old. At some point, she had expressed wanting to get her nose done, so they brought her in for a consultation.

During the consult, I noticed a few things. One was that the girl herself was quite anxious and nervous. She wouldn't make eye contact with me. The parents did the talking, telling me about her. I eventually got her talking a bit and pulled her story out, allowing me to hear more from her perspective, by saying, "You have to tell me what *you* want if you want to even continue this consultation."

When it all started to come out, she basically felt like she was not pretty enough. None of the boys liked her. None of her friends thought she was pretty. But when she first walked in, like I always do, I told her how pretty she was. *You're so gorgeous! You have a beautiful face. I love your eyes. I love your smile.* As we continued to talk, she told me that when I said that to her, it was literally one of the first times someone had openly told her how pretty she was. At that moment, it was something that she felt was hugely impactful. As a result, she chose *not* to have surgery.

About two years later, her mom called to tell me that the conversation that day, coming from an "expert in beauty" (what her daughter calls me), really made something click for the young lady. *If an expert in beauty thinks I'm beautiful, clearly I'm not as bad as I think.* From that day forward, her entire life changed in terms of how she behaved, how she acted, how she carried herself, and even how she did in school. **Everything changed.** All I did was tell her how pretty she was. That's it. She needed some external validation from someone other than her parents, and, happily, I had the opportunity to provide it.

The Journey

Did you know your looks are the least interesting thing about you? Think about it. Are you good friends with anyone because of the way they look? Of course not! You are friends with them because they're funny, smart, or empathetic—or maybe all of those things wrapped into one amazing package—but I am quite certain your best friend's beauty quotient never factored in. Frankly, your looks simply aren't that interesting! **So, why do you feel like your beauty needs to be validated by others?**

As humans, we are naturally inclined to place importance on our physical appearance. It's why we compare ourselves to others in our friend circle or celebrities on magazine covers. We see them, admire them, and start to compare ourselves to them—even to the airbrushed, photoshopped versions. If we don't believe we measure up, our feelings of insecurity about our appearance start to grow.

Yet when someone tells us we're pretty (or handsome), it allays some of that insecurity, at least for a little while. If you're not already validating yourself from within, any external praise you receive wears off pretty quickly, and you can become desperate to get more.

What is truly special and interesting about you is what is inside of you. It isn't something that can be seen in a picture or measured by some artificial beauty standard. When you are able to focus on who you truly are, rather than obsessing over external features, you start to become validated from the inside, and that is far more lasting and important. External praise becomes far less significant in shaping how you view yourself.

When you are able to focus on who you truly are, rather than obsessing over external features, you start to become validated from the inside, and that is far more lasting and important.

In the coming chapters, we will take a closer look at where the external voices that shape our beauty perceptions come from and consider whether they really should have the level of influence they do. We will compare the cultural implications of beauty by examining beauty standards around the world in places like South America, India, Africa, South Korea, the Middle East, as well as the U.S. We'll explore the influence of marketing, advertising, aging, and social media on our perceptions of beauty and fashion. Finally, I'll show you practical changes you can make in your own life to finally see yourself as the beautiful person you already are.

We all already share in the unifying struggle *not* to be ugly. Now it's time to unite on this journey together to identify and filter the voices that shape our perceptions of what it means to be beautiful.

Beauty Notes

* Most perceptions and insecurities
  about how beautiful or ugly
  we are come from a need for
  external validation, versus
  an internal validation and
  appreciation for who we are.
  External validation is related to
  why we want to look a certain
  way; internal validation is more
  about how we feel about ourselves
  when we look in the mirror.

* The problem is that when you
  look into the external world for
  beauty validation, you're always
  being sold. As a result, rarely will
  someone talk to you honestly about
  beauty. Think about it: almost
  everyone you encounter in the
  beauty business is a salesperson.

* What is truly special and interesting about you is what is inside of you. It isn't something that can be seen in a picture or measured by some artificial beauty standard. When you are able to focus on who you truly are, rather than obsessing over external features, you start to become validated from the inside, and that is far more lasting and important. External praise becomes far less significant in shaping how you view yourself.

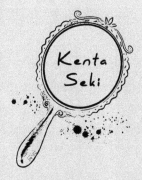

Kenta Seki

As a superstar in the fitness industry, celebrity trainer Kenta Seki is acutely aware of just how much of a role external validation plays in whether a person feels beautiful or not. And while you might think that feeling insecure about appearance is an issue only women struggle with, Kenta knows that's simply not the case.

When he was young, Kenta was, in his words, "super, super skinny." As he got into high school and started being more aware of how his physical appearance compared to others, he became intentional about what he could do to make himself feel more attractive, get more compliments, and (he assumed) be even more well-liked.

At age nine, he began practicing Yoga and really fell in love with it, to the point where at sixteen he even became a Yoga instructor. "Being around all the gym equipment got me interested in general fitness, and I soon became a certified personal trainer as well."

Kenta began really gaining muscle, and as he did, people started complimenting him on his physique more and more frequently. That external validation was definitely a self-esteem booster, as it would be for all of us. But also like all of us, Kenta harbored some self-doubt.

He shares, "The fitness industry can be intimidating. There are so many really fit and good-looking people that it's easy to feel like you're not good enough. At the beginning of my career, I felt like I wasn't as fit as the other trainers at my gym, so I was actually hesitant to get into personal training. Eventually I came to understand that your success as a trainer is actually more about your personality and people skills than it is about your looks."

Kenta has worked with countless clients and has found that men and women, celebrities or not, share that common thread of insecurity about their appearance in some way. Women may think men don't worry about it, but that's just because guys tend to talk about their concerns with other guys instead of with women.

"There is pressure on men to be fit to unattainable standards. It starts young, with characters boys see like Batman, Superman, and other male figures planting the subconscious idea that's what we're supposed to look like. It's unrealistic."

He concedes, "Maybe there isn't as much pressure on men in society to focus on all the little things about their appearance as there is on women. But there's still absolutely some pressure there." Whether it's wanting to lose some weight, uncover a six-pack, or stop the receding hairline, there are plenty of ways guys feel "less than" too.

To combat those voices of doubt, Kenta encourages his clients to look for more internal validation than external validation. "There have been countless times that I've had an injury or something slowed me down to where my body may not have looked or felt the best. I realized, though, that I can't place my sole value on how I look outside, because then I would start to feel terrible about myself.

I've learned to value who I am on the inside more. And it's a lifelong journey; you have to tackle it each time those negative thoughts start to come up. For me, my true purpose is in helping people improve their health and fitness. It's what keeps me going forward, and no matter how I look on the outside, if I'm fulfilling that purpose, then I can feel good about myself."

In addition to living with purpose, Kenta encourages his clients to keep close tabs on that inner voice. "Our thoughts are conversations we have with ourselves—keeping them positive can have a direct influence on our actions and our results.

Do your best to replace negative thoughts with positive ones. Maybe that means being proud that you woke up and got to the gym even if it wasn't your best workout, or feeling confident that you can crush a new fitness class instead of dreading it."

While you might see a photo of Kenta Seki and admire his phenomenal physique, keep in mind that he makes a point of staying internally validated rather than letting the voices of external validation be the only ones to shape his self-worth.

And that's a lesson from him you can get for free!

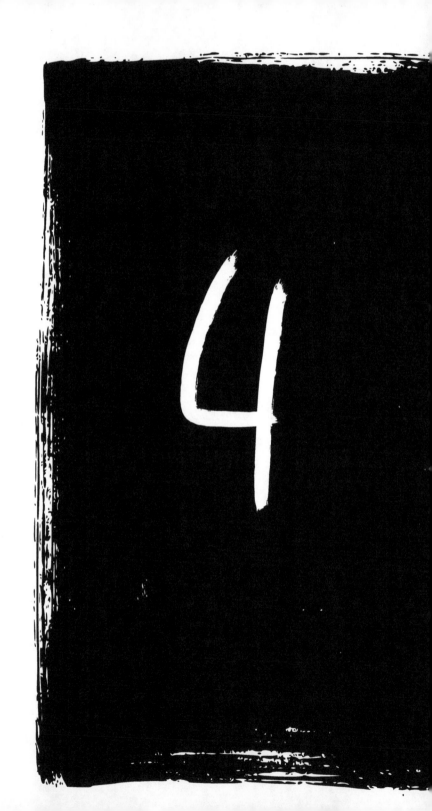

The Voices That Shape Us

Beauty is a matter of perception, plain and simple. Have you ever looked at a flower and admired how beautiful it is? Of course, you have. But while admiring that flower, have you ever broken down the schematic design of that same flower and said because the petals are arranged in a 30-degree ratio from each other, that must be why you considered it beautiful? Of course not, because that would be absurd.

Yet with our own beauty, we have done that. Yes, there has actually been research conducted to try to identify mathematical universal standards of beauty in terms of symmetry. One such study, conducted by the National Institutes of Health, finds that "beautiful faces have ideal facial proportion...and that proportion is 1 to 1.618."[1] Likewise, researchers at the University of California in San Diego and the University of Toronto discovered that "the distance between the centers of a woman's eyes affects whether she is considered beautiful. People find her most attractive when that distance is just under half of the width of the face. Just as important, they found, is the distance between a woman's eyes and mouth. It should be just over one-third the height of her face."[2]

This super nerdy math is what all plastic surgeons are taught in school. Some of my colleagues actually use these ridiculous equations when analyzing faces or during surgery to try to *recreate* beauty. But I tell all my patients that those formulas are nonsense, and true beauty all comes down to *perception*. **What you perceive to be beautiful *is beautiful*...to you.** But the reverse is also true about the perception of ugly. Each of us tries to align with our own perception of beauty; however, many of us fall short of our own perceptions, which leads to feeling ugly, or at least unattractive.

We all
externalize our
perceptions
of beauty
based on
other people's
perceptions of
beauty rather
than actually
internalizing our
own concepts
of beauty.

Perception, however, can be deceiving. We all externalize our perceptions of beauty based on *other people's perceptions* of beauty rather than actually internalizing *our own concepts* of beauty. Have you ever heard a song and couldn't tell if you fully liked it or not? And then you hear your friends or the general popular opinion of the song, and realize *your* opinion of the song became biased based on the popular opinion. We do the same with our perceptions of beauty.

Consider how the perception of beauty has changed throughout history. During the eras of Ancient Greece, the Italian Renaissance, and Victorian England, the "rounder" woman was considered the ideal body shape. The standard of feminine beauty praised by Anglo-Saxon poets of the Middle Ages was a waxy, pale complexion so sought after that some women actually bled themselves regularly to achieve it![3] Because Victorians perceived tiny rosebud lips as the most beautiful, they would consider the full, sensuous mouths admired today to be quite ugly.

Arguably the most prevalent perception of beauty, though, became the Westernized concept propagated through media—film and television, magazines, and now social media. **No matter what part of the**

world you're in, everyone is enamored with Western beauty. If you were left alone in a bubble and never told what other people think beauty is—if you just had to figure it out for yourself—beauty would be defined very differently. But even Western perceptions of beauty have changed through the decades.

In the 1920s, the slim, androgynous look of the flapper was considered beautiful. That gave way to the hourglass figure of the 1930s through the 1950s, only to reappear in the 1960s when models like Twiggy set the beauty standard with her "twiggy" figure, pale lips, and heavily made-up eyes.

The 1970s showcased beauty in terms of the Farrah Fawcett-style suntan, "wings" hairdo, glowing smile, and slim-yet-curvy body. By the 1980s, the beauty standard was big, permed hair with mile-high bangs. Eyeliner and eyeshadow were brightly colored blues and greens, and there was no such thing as "too much makeup." Much like the '70s, beautiful bodies were simultaneously athletic, thin, and curvy.

Even through the present day, perceptions of beauty are always shifting, and anyone who tries to constantly adjust their appearance to always be perceived as beautiful is fighting a losing battle.

Perceptions
of beauty are
always shifting,
and anyone
who tries to
constantly adjust
their appearance
to always be
perceived
as beautiful
is fighting a
losing battle.

Look Who's Talking

Beauty perceptions have been shaped by culture since the beginning of time, really. In turn, culture is shaped a great deal by media in all of its forms, and that's nothing new. According to *Ad Age*, a leading resource on advertising and marketing:

> The first crude advertisements for cosmetics appeared in European newspapers during the 17th and 18th centuries. Powder made of white lead and ground rice was sold by the pound for whitening the skin and hair. Another product advertised was the beauty patch, used primarily to cover the pockmarks left by smallpox and other diseases, as were rouge and lipstick. Early American newspapers featured similar ads, enticing colonists to imitate the latest fashions of London and Paris.[4]

Silent film stars in the early 1900s helped set fashion trends of the time. In fact, Macy's department stores sold duplicates of the gowns worn by the screen stars. Their publicity claimed, "We have disseminated hundreds of Greta Garbos, Joan Crawfords, and Irene Dunnes. We can give almost anyone the cinema glamour."[5]

The first beauty and fashion magazine *Harper's Bazaar* was published on November 2, 1867, claiming to be "a repository of fashion, pleasure, and instruction." More than eighty-five beauty, fashion, and style magazines have been published around the world since then, and no one can argue the role they have in influencing our global perceptions of beauty.

Naturally, television began to shape our beauty perceptions as soon as it became a widespread medium, not only through the beautiful actors and actresses on the programs, but by the advertisements for beauty, fashion, and health products.

Currently, the biggest influence on our beauty perceptions is—you guessed it—social media. A study conducted by British Parliament of over 7,000 people revealed the following unsurprising (yet unfortunate) statistics:

> Under Age 18: Social media is the number one influence over body image. Adults 18 and over: Social media is the number three influence over body image (behind exercise and healthy eating).[6]

One study suggested that 95% of patients considering a cosmetic procedure had consulted an online source, including social media.[7] Other studies evaluating the reasons patients pursue cosmetic procedures cite experiences with social media as a key factor.

In fact, social media has become such a shaping factor in (false) beauty perceptions, I regularly discuss how to filter that voice with my patients. If they are looking at images of stereotypically beautiful people and feel ugly afterward, they need to develop the wherewithal to understand that it affects their energy and self-esteem. Acknowledging the problem is always step one, before you can develop strategies to combat the problem. For example, I encourage them to use the programmed features of social media apps to hide or block any content that brings negative energy to their life.

Voices Closer to Home

But it's not just media and the movie stars, television actors, and social media influencers who shape our beauty perceptions. After culture, the real-life people we hang out with are the biggest influencers on our perceptions of beauty—romantic relationships, friends, and family—usually in that order.

Romantic relationships. These are a huge factor in defining how beautiful you feel and how confident you are. If your special someone tells you you're beautiful, it's obviously going to make you feel good about yourself. Even if you don't think you align with cultural beauty standards, knowing someone you care about thinks you're beautiful will often (though not always) mean more.

Friendships. These relationships are the next most influential in shaping our beauty perceptions. If you're friends with people who are uplifting about how amazing and beautiful and great you are, you likely feel confident and energized being around them. But if you are around people making you more self-conscious about the way you look or dress on a daily basis, this could easily bring your energy and confidence down. For example, if you hang around Sue who is always saying, *Oh, you'd be so cute if you did this...* Would you feel your energy level drop and your anxiety go up about your looks?

That's when you may realize you may need to filter some real-life people from your life and not only on social media! What and who you allow into your headspace is truly important in terms of whether or not you perceive yourself to be beautiful.

Family. These are probably the least influential voices we listen to when it's a positive comment (after all, because she's my mom, she *has* to say I'm beautiful). Paradoxically, though, these voices can be the most influential when it comes to negative comments (even my dad says I'm fat, so I *must* be hideous). Mental health counselors hear stories every day from people whose parents messed up their self-worth and self-image. For that matter, so do I! Healing from our childhood traumas and any damage to our self-esteem is a huge part of growing into the beautiful beings we strive to be. Acknowledging how positive or negative our families may have been, in our perceptions of ourselves is a burden we must all undertake before any healing can begin.

But it is important to remember that whether it's your partner, your friends, or your family, all of their perceptions of beauty were influenced by the perceptions of *their* partners, friends, and families as well. **This is an ongoing cycle of influence over perceptions of beauty that we continue to spread and propagate.** And while the Western cultural ideal of beauty is largely accepted as *the* beauty standard we are all programmed by, there are also unique ways beauty is perceived among different cultures around the world. Examining these differences is helpful for understanding the fluid nature of our perceptions of beauty.

Beauty Notes

* Perception can be deceiving.
  We all externalize our
  perceptions of beauty based
  on other people's perceptions
  of beauty rather than
  actually internalizing our
  own concepts of beauty.

* Perceptions of beauty are
  always shifting, and anyone
  who tries to constantly adjust
  their appearance to always
  be perceived as beautiful is
  fighting a losing battle.

* Beauty perceptions have been shaped by culture since the beginning of time, really. In turn, culture is shaped a great deal by media in all of its forms: magazines, television, movies, and especially social media.

* After culture, the real-life people we hang out with are the biggest influencers on our perceptions of beauty—romantic relationships, friends, and family—usually in that order.

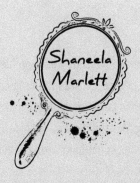

Shaneela
Marlett

Shaneela Marlett is a brilliant attorney, passionate about ensuring Social Security claimants receive their due. After graduating from UCLA with a degree in psychology, she received her Juris Doctorate at Pepperdine University School of Law, where she was the Magister of Phi Delta Phi's Honors Legal Fraternity.

And she's a woman of Pakistani heritage who—just like everyone else—has experienced the feeling that her appearance was somehow lacking, not measuring up to what the world seems to consider beautiful.

Growing up with her single mom, who didn't make a lot of money, she lived in some pretty rough neighborhoods. However, her mom was determined that she would have a great education, so she would take jobs in affluent areas and then use the work address to register Shaneela in "better" schools—but they lacked diversity.

Shaneela recalls, "I would be the only person of color in the whole school. Everyone looked different than me. Their skin was different. Their features were different. I just always felt on the outside."

That feeling of being different was amplified within her extended family, where she was the only one with curly hair. Well-intentioned family members would say, "Oh, don't worry—we'll straighten it when you get older." To Shaneela, that meant there was something wrong with her.

Or she'd hear, "Oh, your nose is from your father's side of the family; it's not our family nose." And again, they'd promise she could fix it when she got older. The seed was planted that she was not quite pretty enough, and that seed continued to grow.

As soon as she turned eighteen, Shaneela had rhinoplasty. (And yes, there are some instances where such a procedure really can make an improvement, which is part of the joy and satisfaction I get when I'm fortunate enough to be able to make that transformation for a patient.) She says, "It was a real self-confidence boost for me, but more superficially. Internally, I still struggled with self-love for many more years."

A few years ago, Shaneela faced some post-partum issues and marital challenges, and her internal struggle with self-image kicked in again. Intellectually, she knew such thinking wasn't rational, but emotionally she couldn't help going there.

She unconsciously lost weight, and she started looking into fillers and other cosmetic procedures. She found herself drawn back to thinking her nose was a problem but was afraid of having surgery again. Her research led her to Scarless Nose™ Rhinoplasty and into my office.

She shares, "I went to see Dr. Dugar and showed him all of these pictures of what I thought my nose could look like. He told me, 'Your nose is perfect. I wouldn't touch it!' It was really surprising to me because here was a doctor who could make a lot of money, but he's just telling me I'm ok!

It meant so much to me, and really made me realize that it's not on the outside; that my perception was something I needed to fix on the inside. So I started working with my therapist, and I really feel so much better.

Sometimes it takes someone to be honest and direct, and to bring it to your awareness that anything you do on the outside isn't going to fix what's on the inside."

Shaneela, with her gorgeous, thick, curly hair and Middle Eastern features, is learning to embrace what truly makes each and every one of us beautiful, and is making sure her two young sons understand that what makes them unique is also what makes them perfect—just the way they are!

5

Beauty Around the World

Do you have an hourglass figure? Congratulations! You have the most beautiful body type...in Brazil. What if you're skinny with a flat chest and narrow hips? Congratulations! You also have the most beautiful body type...in South Korea. And so it goes. Around the world, the perception of what makes someone beautiful changes with geography and culture. Each culture has its own beauty standards. However, in this modern era of rapid, visual communication, we are starting to see a shift from regional cultural beauty perceptions to more widely accepted universal perceptions of beauty.

This homogenous beauty standard is dictated largely by Western culture. For women, it includes features such as round eyes, light skin, thin body, small nose, high cheekbones, and so on, even though women in other cultures may naturally look nothing like that. The end result is different approaches to beauty within individual cultures even as they attempt to align more with the Western culture yet remain slightly distinct.

The Western ideal of beauty (USA, Canada, Western Europe) is the dominant standard to which many around the world aspire. This standard consists of the look so often portrayed in Western media: long hair, light skin, big eyes, a slender frame, and large breasts. British psychotherapist Susie Orbach says, "Just as English has become the *lingua franca* of the world, so the white, blondified, small-nosed, pert-breasted, long-legged body is coming to stand in for the great variety of human bodies that there are."[1] In short, Western beauty perceptions shape how women and girls view themselves by promoting what is really an unattainable beauty standard that does not allow for cultural and individual differences.

Western beauty
perceptions
shape how
women and girls
view themselves
by promoting
what is really
an unattainable
beauty standard
that does not
allow for cultural
and individual
differences.

Studies have shown that attractiveness according to the Western standard is a source of power for women in relationships and careers. These women are less lonely, more popular, more sexually experienced, are more likely to marry, and are more likely to marry men of a higher socioeconomic status. These "beautiful" women are also more likely to get hired, promoted, and paid higher salaries.[2]

Because of the unrelenting pressure on women to align with Western beauty standards and enjoy the apparent benefits, **many women and girls view their physical appearance as a source of distress**. This is not only the case in Western cultures. It has become a global problem.

Perhaps a quick tour of some of these regional approaches will help reveal these shifting global perceptions of beauty and the lengths women go to pursue this artificial standard.

South Korea

One mark of beauty in South Korea is to have a youthful, innocent look that begins with a small face. In general, Asian people—and particularly Korean people—have smaller eyes, which makes the face appear larger. To counter that effect, many Koreans (both women and men) attempt to achieve a v-shaped face with unpronounced jawlines and a pointy chin.

Whereas makeup contouring is often leveraged in Western societies to accentuate cheekbones and jawlines, it is used to diminish them in South Korea. Tools such as chin straps and face rollers are used along with jawline facial masks to firm the skin and lift the jawline. But when that's not enough, or when they have the financial resources to do so, **many Koreans turn to plastic surgery to force their faces to fit the beauty perceptions.**

To achieve the look described above, Koreans undergo a reconstruction of the entire middle face and jaw via orthognathic surgery called double jaw surgery. This procedure was normally indicated only for patients with extremely misaligned teeth. But this extremely invasive technique has now permeated pop culture for cosmetic purposes. It requires the plastic surgeon to access the maxilla in the middle of the face and mandible bone of the jaw and then to cut through them with a saw and actually remove pieces of bone. The surgeon then uses screws and metal plates to reposition the jaw to become smaller and more V-shaped to be more aesthetically pleasing based on the desired look.

This extreme procedure involves a serious risk of injury to major blood vessels and nerves which could cause permanent numbness or even facial paralysis. It causes significant facial swelling to the point that many patients require overnight intubation to protect their airway and allow them to breathe. They will experience one to three months—sometimes even up to six months!—of post-surgical facial swelling. Even with all these risks, it is estimated that **more than 5,000 people in South Korea undergo this procedure annually, and the number increases every year.**

Large eyes are another key part of a youthful appearance, yet most Koreans have small eyes with monolids. Also known as an epicanthic fold, a monolid is a skin fold on the upper eyelid that makes it appear that there is no visible crease line below the brow area. One way people achieve a double eyelid is by using invisible two-sided eyelid tape. They push the tape into the eyelid crease so that when the eye opens, the double eyelid fold is created. (You can easily search for a video online on the process if you're having a hard time imagining it.)

Here again, plastic surgery is another popular option to achieve this eye effect. One procedure, the double eyelid surgery, involves recreating the upper eyelid to have a deeper groove that is naturally present in most non-Asian faces. It starts with removing eyelid skin and repositioning eyelid muscles and ligaments through suturing techniques to recreate a deeper groove of the eyelid. Obviously, there is always the risk of permanent scarring and dryness to the eyes, as well as the worst-case scenario of damage to the eyes themselves.

Contrary to the Western ideal of tanned skin, Koreans prefer to be pale. This is in part due to the social construct of paler skin being associated with high-paying jobs, whereas darker skin is associated with outdoor, manual labor. In addition to sun-screen and UV protective gear, many Koreans use skin-lightening face masks regularly.

Koreans also turn to diets, dieting pills, and plastic surgery to achieve the extremely slim figure that is considered beautiful. Sadly, they have seen a dramatic increase in eating disorders, a trend exacerbated by the skyrocketing popularity of Korean pop music stars or K-pop. As Nancy Matsumoto says in Psychology Today:

> K-pop has been hugely influential in the whole diet scene because people want to look like their favorite K-pop stars. Many of these stars are known for their extreme diets. Popular looks include "chopsticks legs" or "lollipop head," a big head fronted with a cute face and Westernized eyes on top of stick-thin legs."[3]

Unfortunately, that is a textbook description of the appearance of a person who suffers from disordered eating.

All of the features described above represent the extreme effort that many women and men in South

Korea undertake to align with a perception of beauty that goes against what is natural for them.

Middle East

The Middle East is made up of many countries—Saudi Arabia, Turkey, UAE, Palestine, Egypt, Iran, Iraq, Israel, and more. It is important to acknowledge that women in the Middle East have varying degrees of rights and freedom, which means that **sometimes it is not about whether a woman perceives herself as beautiful, but if her husband does**. In many of these cultures, women are expected, and in some cases required, to go to great lengths to appear beautiful to him.

For example, although not directly related to appearance, many Middle Eastern women undergo a hymen repair procedure (hymenoplasty) to ensure their new husband will either "feel a pop" or see blood spots on the sheets on their wedding night. A woman's hymen can be torn in numerous ways other than sexual intercourse, such as cycling, swimming, horseback riding, or even by using tampons. But in some Middle Eastern cultures, it is extremely important for a woman's hymen to be intact on her wedding night. **Some women have been divorced or even killed for not having this perceived evidence of virginity.**

The tragic irony is that the woman may also risk death if anyone in her family or her husband's family finds out that she has had the procedure. According to one doctor who performs hymenoplasty, often in the dark of night, women "frequently give false names and pay in cash. They arrive alone, faces hidden, under elaborate hats, wigs, scarves, and sunglasses, and afraid."[4] These extreme measures indicate the extent to which women will go to conform to perceptions of what they physically *should be*.

In terms of physical beauty, Middle East cultures particularly define it by the face, mostly by the eyes, followed by lips and cheeks. This is in large part due to the fact that across much of the Middle East, women's bodies are entirely covered with traditional cultural clothing. Only certain parts of the face are exposed. A burka, for example, covers the face entirely, with just a mesh screen for the woman to see through. A niqab shows only the eyes, while a hijab shows the entire face.

Middle Eastern women are less likely to attempt to align with traditional Western beauty standards; instead, they attempt to achieve a perfect version of the ideal Middle Eastern standard.

A face that is considered beautiful in this culture is an "oval or round face; large almond-shaped eyes; prominent, elevated, arched eyebrows; a small, straight nose; well-defined, laterally full cheeks; full lips; a well-defined jawline; and a prominent, pointed chin."[5] Middle Eastern women are less likely to attempt to align with traditional Western beauty standards; instead, they attempt to achieve a perfect version of the ideal Middle Eastern standard.

These women tend to feel, or be considered by many men to be, ugly if they perceive their face as too heavy or flat; if their noses are too prominent, too flat and wide, or have the typical Middle Eastern bump or hook; if they have poorly defined jawlines (jowls); if their eyes appear hollow, or if they see their chin as too small. Women in this region typically have more body hair than women from Western cultures. They also work to overcome the natural effects of aging on their appearance.

In the 1980s, plastic surgery started to boom in the region. Because it became cheap, easily accessible, and socially acceptable, more and more people have started seeking surgical intervention for their per-ceived flaws. In fact, in the 1980s, the leader of Iran,

Ayatollah Khomeini, "sanctioned rhinoplasty based on religious grounds; he said that 'God is beautiful and loves beauty.'"[6] Today Dubai has the highest concentration of cosmetic surgeons in the world.

In addition to rhinoplasties, the most common procedure women undergo is a tear trough filler to plump up the hollow under-eye area. This procedure involves injecting some type of augmenting hyaluronic filler to re-volumize the area. There is risk to the vessels and nerves around the eyes, as well as potentially **post-traumatic hydrophilic swelling that can last months or even years.**

The Middle Eastern standard of beauty has gained popularity in Western culture in recent years due in part to celebrities like the Kardashian sisters and other notable beautiful women such as Queen Rania Al-Abdullah of Jordan.

Latin America

In Latin America, the beauty ideal focuses on a blend of both Hispanic and Western features, including lightly tanned and hairless skin, long hair, large light-colored eyes, plump lips, and a curvy hourglass figure. Manicured nails and minimal, natural-looking makeup are also part of women's beauty routines. **In Brazil, beauty *is* the culture.** Being perceived as beautiful is considered critical not only for attracting a partner, but also even for getting a good job.

Brazilian women in particular are expected to have a toned and curvy bottom half and often feel extreme pressure to look perfect in a bikini. Butt implants or fat injections are commonplace in Brazil and other areas of Latin America. The procedure has even been nicknamed around the world the "Brazilian Butt Lift." It starts with vacuum-assisted liposuction, which uses a metal cannula (straw-like tube) to suck out fat from different parts of the body—abdomen, flanks, upper arms, or upper back—and reinject that same fat back into the body along the buttocks and thighs to make the area rounder and tighter, much like filling a balloon.

This is one of the most high-risk surgical procedures of all the procedures I've mentioned so far, with the most devastating risk being a fat embolism. If the surgeon penetrates one of the larger blood vessels in the buttocks area while injecting the fat, a piece of fat can make its way inside of the vessel and travel to the lungs, potentially killing the patient.

An alternative to the fat injection is the use of silicone implants in the buttocks. It works in a way that is similar to breast implants. It was most popular in the 1980s and '90s but is still occasionally used today.

Lymphatic drainage massage is another beauty process to reduce swelling and eliminate toxins that is popular among Brazilian women to help achieve the body they desire. This process involves bringing the fluid stuck in between cells and in tissue to the lymph nodes in order to be pumped out of the body. The procedure, according to Joanna Vargas, celebrity facialist and salon owner, "involves the whole body and begins by stimulating the lymph nodes, starting from the pelvic area, the groin, under the knees and ankles, armpits, collar bone, and most importantly, the thoracic duct. It uses soft pressure, to encourage a healthy lymph flow through a series of strokes and patterns along the lymphatic pathway."[7]

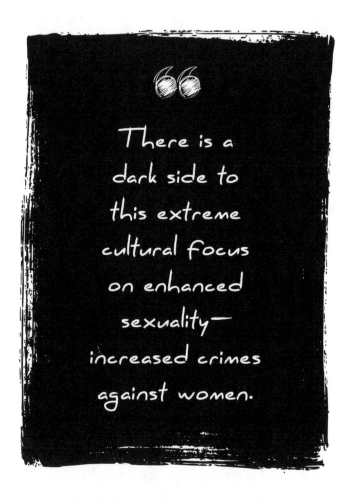

There is a dark side to this extreme cultural focus on enhanced sexuality—increased crimes against women.

As a result of this focus on beauty, Brazil is known for its beautiful women. They are number one in the world for both breast and butt augmentation procedures; however, there is a dark side to this extreme cultural focus on enhanced sexuality—increased crimes against women. Brazilians even call it the "cultura do estupro" which means "rape culture" in Portuguese. In 2018 alone, Brazil registered more than 66,000 cases of sexual violence, more than 180 rapes per day.[8] Many organizations campaign to end all forms of violence against women and girls, including sexual and other types of exploitation, but there is still a long way to go.[9]

India

The Indian perception of beauty is strongly correlated with skin color. In fact, a woman could be considered beautiful only if she were "Gori" (white or fair) and had no specific deformities.[10] Many believe this colorism is tied to India's colonization by the British Empire, but in fact, Aryans came into India from Europe and Central Asia nearly 2000 years BCE. They were naturally fairer than the native people. As they assumed ruling, a version of white supremacy began.[11]

Even today, being fair represents having wealth, luxury, and status. Maybelline is a global makeup brand that offers forty shades of foundation elsewhere in the world so women can find a close match to their skin tone. It only offers seventeen shades in India, mostly light shades—because that is what the consumers have been conditioned to believe is beautiful.[12]

Advertisements show fair women are happier and more successful, furthering the idea that life is tough if you have darker skin. One dermatologist notes that more than half of her clients each day come to her for skin-lightening procedures.[13] Well-known fairness brands in India sell fairness cream, lotion, face wash, deodorants, and even a vaginal whitener to the tune of $4 billion per year and growing.[14]

After targeting the female audience for years, advertisers have moved on to males and even babies. A commercial for Healthy and Fair baby massage oil announces it "makes your baby strong with a pink fairness" and shows a baby becoming lighter and then holding a trophy and wearing a crown, as if winning a baby beauty pageant.[15]

Outside of skin color, the Indian beauty standard also includes large eyes, a narrow waist with wider hips, long, black, thick, wavy hair, and full red lips. Before the influence of Western beauty standards,

Indians historically preferred women with curvy, hourglass figures and even a bit of a belly pooch. Now, slim figures are more often seen as a beauty indicator. This is not necessarily a bad thing, because it has brought an increased focus on fitness and health that didn't really exist before.

But there is the other side of the coin. Eating disorders were nominal in Indian culture as recently as the 1990s, but Indian psychiatrists have noted that in the past decade, the number of Indian women suffering from disordered eating has increased between five and ten times. It is also impacting women at younger ages.[16] According to Ruchi Anand, American Graduate School professor of International Relations, "Now what we're seeing is a trend toward an imitation of the Westernized body image. These girls literally are fighting for the size zero, which was never known as beautiful in India."[17]

While fashion plays a part in the perception of beauty in virtually every culture (we'll dive deeper into that topic later), it is especially important in Indian culture. The way Indian people wear clothing is related to their social status and education level. Traditional Indian dress varies by region with differences in how a woman's sari or man's dhoti is wrapped or the cut of the design. The use of a head-dress or hairdressing, or the use of temporary or permanent body markings and jewelry align with caste, religious, regional, or ethnic identity.[18]

It comes as no surprise that body image issues are rampant among Indian girls. Such issues are unfor-tunately often exacerbated by the negative influence of family members or friends, as appearance is fair game for conversation among Indian families.

Blogger Varsha Patel shared the following story about her experience growing up:

> Eyebrows need to be thick but shapely. Skin needs to be clear and glowing, not to mention fair. Hair must be long, lus-cious, thick, and undyed. No bob cuts under any circumstances. Nose pierc-ings? Okay. But not on the wrong side. It must be on the Indian side...

An open, healthy discussion about beauty and feeling comfortable in my own skin never formed part of my growing up. My white friends could talk to their parents about their skin problems, for example, but as a 13-year-old, my family told me "fine natee lagtu" ("this doesn't look nice") followed by the ground-breaking advice: "Just go to the doctor."[19]

And go to the doctor they do. **India ranks fifth in the world in plastic surgery with nearly 900,000 procedures annually.**[20]

Africa

Beauty standards in Africa are widely varied with everything from the Middle Eastern standards of many North African countries to the tribal standards of the Maasai, Himba, Zulu, and others around central and South Africa. For our purposes here, I'll focus on the tribal beauty standards, though even those vary from one cultural community to another. Notably, these tribal cultures do *not* make an effort to align with the Western beauty standard; rather, they are very distinctly their own.

There are some differences in beauty standards that are unique to this area of the world. For one, beauty is seen as a union of physical attractiveness and good manners or conduct; in other words, **a combination of inner and outer beauty**. A person can be considered lacking in beauty who is missing one of the halves of that combination.

In general, youthfulness, skin hues (yellow or red), and full faces tend to predict what is considered attractive in African female faces. Heavier women are considered attractive in traditional African tribal culture because low body weight can be seen as an indicator of illness and disease.

Tribal marks are also a large part of what is considered beautiful. These marks differ between tribes as a means of identification, and they differ in shape, size, and location. In the past, these marks were made with knives (thereby scarring the skin), but that practice has been abolished and replaced with tattooing or face painting with clay. Different colors of paint have different symbols in each community.

Other tribal practices include creating long ear-lobes with heavy jewelry and stretching the bottom lip by making a hole in the lip and inserting wooden or clay plates. Dreadlocks are a popular hairstyle worn by many cultures across Africa. This style is believed to have originated from the Maasai tribe in Kenya, spreading to other parts of Africa and then across the globe. Teeth chiseling—creating sharp points—is a beauty practice of the Afar tribe in Ethiopia, marking a young girl's passage into womanhood.

A high forehead is a beauty ideal among the Fula tribe in Nigeria, so those born without it will remove parts of their hair from their heads to achieve the look. Meanwhile, the beauty standard among women of the Samburu tribe in Kenya is to shave their hair altogether, and then show off their shaved heads by wearing layers of colorful beaded necklaces. And while it's not technically observable beauty, tribal men of the Hadza tribe in Tanzania prefer women who don't bathe, since extreme body odor is considered beautiful.[22]

Fashion plays a major role in African tribal beauty as well. Tribes have unique dresses that they wear for ceremonies or special occasions. **The type of garment used for their clothing represents their status in the community and symbolizes ethnic group, tribal allegiance, status, or special ritual.** They use brightly colored printed fabrics as wraparounds for their bodies. Accessories include belts, caps, bags, and headdresses made of seashells, beads, furs, or animal tails. Even outside of tribes, in the more modern cities, African women still wear traditional dresses, but they use them for everyday wear rather than just special occasions.

Arguably one reason these African tribes remain relatively unaffected by Western influence is that they are not exposed to media and advertising as widely as other cultures. More than half of sub-Saharan Africans don't have electricity[23], so they're certainly not seeing television advertisements, nor are they scrolling through social media on computers. They're not picking up copies of *Vogue* or *People Magazine*.

In fact, looking at how little these people are influenced by Western beauty standards really puts a spotlight on just how influential media of all sorts can be.

Beauty Notes

* Around the world, the perception of what makes someone beautiful changes with geography and culture. Each culture has its own beauty standards. However, in this modern era of rapid, visual communication, we are starting to see a shift from regional cultural beauty perceptions to more widely accepted universal perceptions of beauty.

* The Western ideal of beauty (USA, Canada, Western Europe) is the dominant standard to which many around the world aspire. This standard consists of the look so often portrayed in Western media: long hair, light skin, big eyes, a slender frame, and large breasts.

* Western beauty perceptions
  shape how women and girls view
  themselves by promoting what
  is really an unattainable beauty
  standard that does not allow for
  cultural and individual differences.

6

You Are Being Sold

How many ads do you think you see each day? 100? 500? Before you answer, consider everywhere you are exposed to advertising and marketing.

* Do you listen to the radio?
* Scroll through social media?
* See billboards or signs when you drive?
* Watch television?
* Shop anywhere?
* Read magazines or newspapers?

And those are just advertisements. Now think of all of the times each day you're exposed to marketing via brand labels: food, clothing, shoes, makeup, and more.

It's not surprising then that **the average person is exposed to 4,000 to 10,000 ads per day!**[1] Most of the time it doesn't even consciously register or, if it does, we think we're immune. In her book *Can't Buy My Love: How Advertising Changes the Way We Think and Feel*, Jean Kilbourne notes:

> The fact is that much of advertising's power comes from this belief that advertising does not affect us. The most effective kind of propaganda is that which is not recognized as propaganda. Because we think advertising is silly and trivial, we are less on guard, less critical, than we might otherwise be. It's all in fun; it's ridiculous. While we're laughing, sometimes sneering, the commercial does its work.[2]

This is especially true in the beauty industry. When we see an advertisement for a beauty product, even if we don't consciously register it, the ad is doing its work. It is making us feel somehow less beautiful, maybe even a little bit bad about how we look.

When we see an
advertisement for
a beauty product,
even if we
don't consciously
register it, the
ad is doing its
work. It is making
us feel somehow
less beautiful,
maybe even a little
bit bad about
how we look.

We don't even have to see an airbrushed, photo-shopped model, just seeing the products will do the trick. The *Journal of Consumer Research* found that "exposure to beauty-enhancing products in adver-tisement lowered consumers' self-evaluations in much the same way as exposure to thin and attrac-tive models in advertisements has been found to lower self-evaluations."[3] So what do we do? **We subconsciously start to think we need to pur-chase something to make us more beautiful.** Our insecurities are being fed whether we realize it or not.

Cosmetics

According to Harvard Health, the average woman uses many different categories of beauty products every day, including shampoos and conditioners, hair dyes, fragrances, skincare products (cleansers, toners, serums, moisturizers, etc.), body lotions, sunscreen, nail polish, and makeup. Each of those categories contains multiple products—a typical woman's makeup drawer contains at least forty dif-ferent products![4]

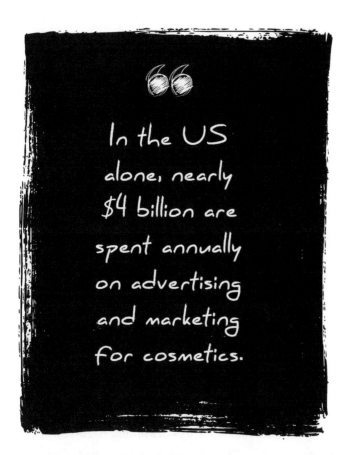

> In the US alone, nearly $4 billion are spent annually on advertising and marketing for cosmetics.

That is why the global cosmetics industry is enormous, grossing hundreds of billions of dollars each year and **expected to top *half a trillion* dollars per year by 2027.**[5] In the US alone, nearly $4 billion dollars are spent annually on advertising and marketing for cosmetics.

What message are they sending? Consider one well-known slogan: "Maybe she's born with it; maybe it's Maybelline." This catchy phrase implies that if you don't feel naturally beautiful, like you're born with it (and statistically most women don't), then Maybelline cosmetics can help make you look more beautiful.

Apparently, it's working. Maybelline is one of the best-selling makeup brands worldwide.[6] Just remember, though, Maybelline is selling to you, just like every other makeup brand out there. While their secondary purpose is to build your self-confidence, **the primary purpose of their marketing is to keep you feeling like you're not your best self** unless you're using their cosmetics. Their ultimate goal as a company is to make money—Maybelline generates nearly $150 million in annual sales. And that is a drugstore brand. High-end cosmetics, like Chanel, routinely top $10 billion in annual revenue.[7]

In the UK, the Advertising Standards Authority (ASA) acts as a watchdog over advertising which can be misleading or irresponsible. Several years ago, a Maybelline ad for an anti-aging product featuring model Christy Turlington was banned. The ad showed parts of the model's face covered by the foundation while other parts were not, supposedly showing how well the product worked to erase fine lines. The company later admitted that Turlington's image had been "digitally retouched to lighten the skin, clean up makeup, reduce dark shadows and shading around the eyes, smooth the lips and darken the eyebrows."[8]

British politician, Jo Swinson, filed a complaint about the ad:

> Pictures of flawless skin and super-slim bodies are all around, but they don't reflect reality… Excessive airbrushing and digital manipulation techniques have become the norm, but Christy Turlington doesn't need retouching to look great. This ban sends a powerful message to advertisers–let's get back to reality.[9]

If it sounds like I'm picking on Maybelline, you can insert any well-known makeup brand in their place. In one instance, L'Oreal was sued when experts recognized that actress Kate Moss was wearing false eyelashes in an ad promoting a lash lengthening mascara to consumers. L'Oreal marketed the product claiming that it would improve lash length by as much as 60%.[10] Nope. It was the false eyelashes, which anyone can purchase at a drugstore for a few dollars, that added the length.

I'm also not picking on makeup in general. **Most women really do feel more confident with a little lipstick, blush, or mascara—and that's great!** My concern is simply that you should buy it because you like the quality of the product, or the color choices, or whatever criteria is important to you—not because you believe you will experience a miraculous transformation to align with false standards of beauty being sold to you through marketing.

Fashion

Cosmetics is not the only industry selling us artificial beauty standards and making huge profits; **the**

global fashion market is worth nearly \$1.5 trillion in retail sales each year. If you add in shoes and jewelry, that number rises over \$2 trillion. Those companies pay a great deal to make sure you get the message that fashion matters to your beauty with over \$500 billion spent annually on fashion advertising and marketing.[11]

You may not immediately think you have been influenced by fashion advertising, but think again. If you're of a certain age, you'll probably remember when the 16-year-old and gorgeous Brooke Shields confessed, "Nothing comes between me and my Calvins!" That fashion advertisement has gone down in history as one of the most recognizable (and sexiest) campaigns in fashion history. And if you remember that commercial, you probably also had— or wanted to have—a pair of Calvin Klein jeans. (If you don't remember it, just Google it!)

Abercrombie and Fitch, Tommy Hilfiger, Ralph Lauren, Guess, Gap, Donna Karan—all of these brands and more advertise with young, beautiful models, subtly implying that we will be just as beautiful if we wear their brands. But here's something you may not have known: some of those model depictions are actually made up of parts and pieces of different models to achieve the allegedly perfect look. In 2011, for example, the fashion retailer H&M was busted for pasting models' heads onto computer-generated bodies![12] Let that sink in. **Is what you see in advertising even real?**

I know, you are smart and know that you're too savvy to be affected by such manipulative advertising, but do you have any of those clothing brands in your closet? Do you own any items of clothing you have literally never worn in public, but purchased because of how good it looked online or in the store? If you were presented with two identical shirts or dresses, literally indistinguishable from one another, and one had a name-brand tag on it, which would you choose?

There is
always some
manipulation of
our minds at
play in fashion,
and being
aware of it is
important to
regaining our
authority on
our concepts
of beauty.

There is always some manipulation of our minds at play in fashion, and being aware of it is important to regaining our authority on our concepts of beauty. A few years ago, in a bizarre case of trying to merge fashion and weight loss, several fashion brands marketed shoes that supposedly would help you lose weight and tone your legs just by wearing them. Skechers settled a $40 million lawsuit rather than appear in court when the Federal Trade Commission (FTC) brought suit against them for false claims. Reebok did the same for $25 million. The manufacturers of these shoes had advertised the fitness results without having any proof. Outside testing proved the shoes had zero impact on calorie burning or toning.[13]

Just as with cosmetics, I suggest you **choose for yourself** when it comes to fashion choices. Wear whatever makes *you* feel beautiful. Choose your fashion because of the color, the style, the fabric—not because some company tells you that you'll be more beautiful if you do.

Diet Products

In a world where nearly 25,000 people die from hunger and related causes each day and more than 850 million people are undernourished, it is almost shocking to realize how much money is spent by people looking to lose weight and align with the global beauty standard of thinness. **In the US alone, the weight loss market exceeds $72 billion.**[14,15] The global market will have reached nearly $270 billion by 2024. It's difficult to measure how much is spent on advertising weight loss products each year, but we know that over $400 million has been spent annually just on television advertising for diet programs like Jenny Craig, NutriSystem, and Weight Watchers.[16] Jenny Craig alone spent $34 million in advertising in one recent year.

One study of five women's fitness magazines over a six-month period revealed eighty-seven advertisements for weight loss products. 46% of those advertisements promoted weight loss pills. Another 14% advertised so-called "fat-burners." This same study noted that "weight loss products account for the highest proportion of fraud claims to the FTC.... According to Consumer Reports, 'Since 2010, the FTC

has collected nearly $107 million in consumer resti-
tution for deceptive weight-loss claims.'"[17] **It seems
everyone is looking for a quick-fix miracle
product that will make them look thin.**

Companies looking to profit from people's insecurity
about their weight are quick to exploit the arbitrary
beauty standard of thinness in their advertising. The
Federal Trade Commission has called out some of
the false promises you'll often see in weight-loss ads:

✳ Lose weight without dieting or exercising.
  (You won't.)
✳ You don't have to watch what you eat to lose
  weight. (You do.)
✳ If you use this product, you'll lose weight
  permanently. (Wrong.)
✳ To lose weight, all you have to do is take this
  pill. (Not true.)
✳ You can lose 30 pounds in 30 days. (Nope.)
✳ This product works for everyone. (It doesn't.)
✳ Lose weight with this patch or cream.
  (You can't.)[18]

The weight loss
industry can
be sneaky and
disguise their
marketing as news
stories complete
with testimonials
(made up)
and dramatic
before-and-
after pictures
(photoshopped).

At least when you watch a commercial or see an advertisement, you generally recognize that you're being sold to. The weight loss industry can be sneaky, though, and disguise their marketing as news stories complete with testimonials (made up) and dramatic before-and-after pictures (photoshopped).

An interesting experiment was conducted where a group of women was led to a waiting room where they remained alone for several minutes. The waiting room held two kinds of magazines: health magazines and news magazines. The room also had a table with two kinds of food on it: healthy food and junk food. The women were invited to help themselves to snacks while they waited. The researchers recorded which magazines were read as well as which foods were consumed and how much of each.

The result of the experiment was that participants who perused the health magazine and were exposed to idealized images of beauty ate significantly less junk food than the participants who read the news magazine and the control group. The conclusion was that **exposure to advertisements and images such as these can negatively influence a**

woman's body image, mood, and self-esteem. As a result, those participants opted for eating something they perceived would help them look more beautiful.[19]

Maybe you're thinking that you don't fall for that. You don't buy anything without reading the reviews. The reality is that if you see a too-good-to-be-true product with mostly five-star reviews, the reviews could be fictitious as well. A healthy dose of skepticism should accompany any reviews you read. All it takes is someone with a computer and a bank of names to type up a hundred reviews on their product website and make it look as if they're selling the miracle of all miracle products.

Women and men come in all shapes and sizes and can certainly be beautiful no matter what the scales say. Obviously, separate from the beauty conversation, there are health considerations when it comes to weight. If your weight exceeds healthy levels, it's a good idea to address that. Just don't fall for the advertising and marketing of the get-thin-quick products.

The best way to get yourself healthy is really never advertised at all because long-term dedication and commitment to a healthy diet, exercise regimen, and lifestyle don't make for quick sales and profit!

Plastic Surgery

Yes, even plastic surgeons advertise their services, so I recognize that by writing this in some ways I am calling myself out. If someone wants—and is a good candidate for—rhinoplasty, then I want them to know about me. So, of course, I market and advertise my practice.

A plastic surgeon will typically spend between $60,000 and $200,000 annually on marketing, depending on the size of the practice. There are around 7,000 plastic surgeons in the US, but other specialists such as dermatologists, ophthalmologists, and oral surgeons also offer cosmetic surgical procedures, so it's difficult to nail down a cumulative dollar figure for advertising money spent. Whatever that number is, the result is that **globally nearly $40 billion dollars are spent by men and women each year on cosmetic procedures**. That amount is constantly growing.[20]

Until 1982, the American Medical Association prohibited physicians from advertising procedures.
Then the Supreme Court ruled that this ban was
unlawful. The American Society of Plastic Surgeons
Code of Ethics requires that members' marketing
not include any statement or claim that "appeals
primarily to layperson's fears, anxieties, or emotional vulnerabilities."[21] Think about it, though.
Isn't anyone considering plastic surgery somewhat
emotionally vulnerable about their appearance? In
effect, that's not a very enforceable standard.

In many ways, those in the market for cosmetic procedures are getting younger, and ads are starting
to target them. The widespread use of Snapchat,
the social media site primarily used by a younger
crowd, has led to what is now called "Snapchat
Dysmorphia." It is a term for the unrealistic standards of beauty young people develop as a result of
viewing themselves through Snapchat filters.

I'm sure that I'm not the only plastic surgeon who
has had young people bring filtered or edited photos
of themselves requesting procedures to make them
look more like the edited images. One marketing
company that caters to plastic surgeons even advises

on their website, "Don't miss out on the opportunity to reach out to this younger and more looks-conscious crowd."[22]

While I'm not opposed to operating on a young person, just like with any potential patient, **there has to be a legitimate reason to do the surgery**. Recently a young lady of just sixteen came with her parents all the way to Beverly Hills from Paris for a consultation about a nose job. Her nose looked perfectly fine. She was a pretty girl with no real issues at all, but because of the external messaging she was hearing from social media and from her friends who were having procedures, she thought she needed to do something, too.

When I declined her, she was disappointed and upset. I think her parents were a little confused, too, that I was saying no to the procedure. She said it was my job to do that procedure if she wanted it and was willing to pay for it. Of course, I let her know that my job is actually to do what is right and best for my patients, and it would not be right nor best to alter her nose. Did she go somewhere else and get it done? Maybe. I hope not, but unfortunately, the reality is that not every plastic surgeon in the world thinks as

I do. If they did, there wouldn't be as much market-ing designed to prey on a young girl's insecurities.

Anyone considering plastic surgery should do their research and look much deeper than shiny advertisements or websites. When it comes to cosmetic surgery advertising, appearances can indeed be deceiving.

Influencers

New research shows that influencers like the Kardashian sisters, Mia Kahlifa, Zoe Sugg, Michelle Phan, Kandee Johnson, Huda Kattan, and others have had a significant influence on marketing in the beauty industry. They attract loyal followings on social media with "tribes" of fans who trust these influencers and their recommendations more than they trust traditional media advertisements.

As a result, **even many longtime players in the beauty market are starting to seek partner-ships with influencers.** In fact, cosmetic giant Estée Lauder, which owns at least twenty-seven major brands including Clinique, Aveda, MAC, and the ultra-expensive LaMer, revealed that the company is now spending 75% of its marketing budget on influencers.[23]

In a recent Harvard Business School study of 520 women, 62% said they follow beauty influencers on social media. When they were asked where they seek information about beauty products prior to purchasing them, their sources were social media influencers (67% of the time), third-party product reviews (59%), beauty professionals (55%), brand advertisements (44%), and finally public figures and celebrities at just 34%[24].

Influencer marketing informs their purchasing decisions most, even though they are well aware that brands often pay influencers to promote their products. Many of the respondents said they only follow influencers who openly disclose their endorsement deals. Because consumers seek out influencers who share similar beauty issues (such as skin concerns), they want to trust that influencers they follow actually use and are happy with the products they talk about.[25]

'Kim Kardashian promotes all kinds of products all the time that I'm skeptical she uses,' one consumer said. 'She'll post an Instagram holding a jar of Olay, for example, but then you'll read an interview where she says she always uses a $1,000 Guerlain cream. A celebrity putting their name on something isn't really enough to draw me in by itself.'[26]

When you think of the term *influencers*, you generally think of celebrities or other micro-influencers with huge followings on social media. But you have other influencers in your social media feeds, inbox, and text messages, too—**your friends who are involved in multi-level marketing companies (MLMs)** selling beauty products from skincare to weight loss to supplements and everything in between.

How many times have you had a random text message from an old high school friend just "checking in to see how you're doing" and then telling you all about the life-changing product she has started using? Or maybe you've noticed that suddenly your neighbor no longer posts photos of her kids and pets, but now every post is about the amazing new mascara she's using that quadruples the length of her lashes—and *oh, by the way, you can get it, too*!

Can you trust these friends and their marketing? Maybe. I refer you back to the title of this chapter: understand that *you are being sold*. MLMs provide marketing copy to their members, so most of the time what they are posting isn't even their own words. Look out, again, for the too-good-to-be-true claims and even the "recommended by this doctor", "doctor-approved", or "doctor-tested" endorsements. All it means is one doctor (and maybe even a resident in training!) at some point was paid to put their name on the product endorsement.

If you want to try a product that a celebrity or influencer markets, go ahead. If you want to support your friend in their MLM business, great. Do it. But in every case, realize that the goal of the person pitching the product, whether it's a Kardashian or your next-door neighbor, is not to truly help you be "more" of anything.

The goal is to sell the product and put "more" in their own bank account.

End of story.

The Bottom Line

Suppose you were downtown in a big metropolitan city, late at night, walking by yourself. As you walk down the street, you would be aware of any potential threats around you. You would be hyper-alert that someone could be coming up behind you, lurking in the shadowy doorway just ahead, or hiding in the alleyway ready to jump out.

It may sound overly dramatic, but consuming media advertisements in any form—television commercials, magazine ads, social media posts—can be as dangerous to your self-perception as a dark city street can be to your physical safety. What's worse is that if you're not hyper-alert to it, **you can walk away feeling so much worse about yourself and not even understand why**.

It may sound overly dramatic, but consuming media advertisements in any form—television commercials, magazine ads, social media posts—can be as dangerous to your self-perception as a dark city street can be to your physical safety.

There's a scene in the popular movie *The Devil Wears Prada* where Miranda, the fashion mogul (played by Meryl Streep) who runs the magazine, lectures her fashion-challenged new assistant about why she chose a particular sweater:

> You go to your closet and you select out, oh I don't know, that lumpy blue sweater, for instance, because you're trying to tell the world that you take yourself too seriously to care about what you put on your back. But what you don't know is that that sweater is not just blue, it's not turquoise, it's not lapis, it's actually cerulean.

You're also blithely unaware of the fact that in 2002, Oscar de la Renta did a collection of cerulean gowns. And then I think it was Yves St Laurent, wasn't it, who showed cerulean military jackets? And then cerulean quickly showed up in the collections of eight different designers. Then it filtered down through the department stores and then trickled on down into some tragic "Casual Corner" where you, no doubt, fished it out of some clearance bin. However, that blue represents millions of dollars and countless jobs and so it's sort of comical how you think that you've made a choice that exempts you from the fashion industry when, in fact, you're wearing the sweater that was selected for you by the people in this room.[27]

Why did you choose the lipstick you wear? Why did you choose the shoes you have on today? Why do you have an assortment of face creams in your bath-room drawer? Why are there metabolism-boosting supplements in the medicine cabinet? **You probably don't consciously realize why, but the answer is that you were sold.**

For the next twenty-four hours, pay attention to every single time you are marketed to. Look at every advertisement you see. Notice every billboard. Observe how product placement in the cosmetic aisles draws your attention to certain products.

Try to analyze what the advertisements, commercials, or social media posts are actually trying to do—how they're trying to make you feel. What techniques are they using to do so? Do they subtly promote artificial, unnatural, and impossible beauty standards? Look at the models in the burger commercials or the beer ads. Do you really think they actually eat and drink that way and still look the way they do? Do you think LeBron James, an elite athlete, makes the sugary soft drink that Sprite named after him a big part of his daily diet? I dare you to pay attention, just for one day. I bet it will be eye-opening for you.

Then the next time you feel compelled to purchase anything designed to make you feel or look "better" in some way, think about *why* you feel like you need it and whether you've been sold on the idea that you *need it.*

Beauty Notes

* It's not surprising then that the
  average person is exposed to
  4,000 to 10,000 ads per day!
  Most of the time it doesn't even
  consciously register or, if it does,
  we think we're immune. But
  when we see an advertisement
  for a beauty product, even if
  we don't consciously register
  it, the ad is doing its work. It is
  making us feel somehow less
  beautiful, maybe even a little
  bit bad about how we look.

* Cosmetics, Fashion, and Diet
  Industries spend many billions
  of dollars each year globally on
  advertising. Even plastic surgeons
  advertise, but the American Society
  of Plastic Surgeons Code of Ethics

requires that members' marketing
not include any statement or
claim that "appeals primarily
to layperson's fears, anxieties,
or emotional vulnerabilities."

* In a recent Harvard Business
School study of 520 women, 62%
said they follow beauty influencers
on social media. When they were
asked where they seek information
about beauty products prior to
purchasing them, they listed these
influencers as their first source
more than two-thirds of the time.

* Consuming media advertisements
in any form—television
commercials, magazine ads,
social media posts—can be
as dangerous to your self-
perception as a dark city street
can be to your physical safety.

7

Overexposed: The Social Media Smokescreen

Let's time travel for a moment, back to the '80s, '90s, or even early 2000s—before Mark Zuckerberg released his world-changing software known as Facebook. Imagine you are a high school girl at that time (maybe you actually were!). You have insecurities about your appearance, just like everyone else. You have an idea of what it means to be beautiful based on input you receive from television, movies, and magazines.

You experiment with makeup and fashion, trying to look as cute as the so-called popular girls, who are trying to look as cute as their favorite celebrities and fashion models, who are all trying to align with the beauty standard of the day.

You head to school where perhaps your friends tell you how awesome you look, or a mean girl makes fun of how you look, or nobody mentions your looks at all. At most, you might have five people comment on your appearance one way or another. You go home, watch some TV, flip through a magazine, call your friends, and then do it all again the next day.

Now, fast forward, and imagine you're a present-day teen. Just like the teens of earlier decades, you have insecurities about your appearance. You have an idea of what it means to be beautiful based on the input you receive from television, movies, and magazines, but now your perceptions are supercharged by a new tool—*social media*.

Now you spend hours scrolling through Instagram posts of impossibly beautiful (and likely filtered or air-brushed) people; you watch countless makeup tutorials on YouTube or TikTok; you try dozens of Snapchat filters to see what you'd look like if *this* or *that* were different.

Before you leave for school, you take a handful of selfies until you find one that has just the right angle, lighting, and filters to showcase your outfit, then post it to your stories and head out the door. When you get to the bus stop, you open your phone to discover you already have over 500 likes and dozens of "You look so cute! Love you!" comments. By the time you get to homeroom, you're excited to see that number has doubled.

On the other hand, maybe you get to the bus stop and find you've only had twenty-five people like the photo. And only your best friend commented—so you immediately delete the post and feel bad about yourself all day. You wonder what's wrong with your look that *only* a couple of dozen people liked it! You might even experience the worst-case scenario and have trolls hating on the outfit and posting nasty, snarky comments about how ugly you are and asking why in the world you would even think of going out in public.

Social media has dramatically multiplied— by many thousandfold—the number of voices we let shape our perception of beauty. As a result, the personal dissatisfaction that we feel with regard to our own beauty has skyrocketed.

The Social Data

According to a 2021 Pew Research Study, 70% of Americans now use social media.[1] That number was only 5% in 2005. It increased to 50% in 2011. Take a look at how these numbers break down in the graphic below.

	Facebook	Instagram	Snapchat	YouTube	TikTok
Total	69%	40%	25%	81%	21%
Men	61%	36%	22%	82%	17%
Women	77%	44%	28%	80%	24%
Ages 18-29	70%	71%	65%	95%	48%
30-49	77%	48%	24%	91%	22%
50-64	73%	29%	12%	83%	14%
65+	50%	13%	2%	49%	4%
White	67%	35%	23%	79%	18%
Black	74%	49%	26%	84%	30%
Hispanic	72%	52%	31%	85%	31%
Less than $30K	70%	35%	25%	75%	22%
$30K-$49,999	76%	45%	27%	83%	29%

	Facebook	Instagram	Snapchat	YouTube	TikTok
$50K-$74,999	61%	39%	29%	79%	20%
More than $75K	70%	47%	28%	90%	20%
High school or less	64%	30%	21%	70%	21%
Some college	71%	44%	32%	86%	24%
College graduate	73%	49%	23%	89%	19%

No matter how you break it down, the statistics speak clearly: social media has an enormous shaping impact on our mindset. We know it profoundly impacts everyone's perceptions of beauty. It's not going anywhere, though, so the best line of defense is first to **be aware of its impact**. Even if you don't have a single social media account (which statistically is highly unlikely) and think you're not affected by social media, you are—because everyone around you is being influenced by social media, and you are influenced by those people.

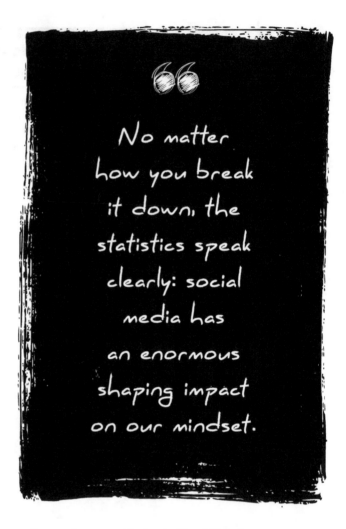

> No matter how you break it down, the statistics speak clearly: social media has an enormous shaping impact on our mindset.

I'm not immune; I'm basically addicted to Instagram. I find myself opening it for no reason. I probably do it because I'm addicted to the motion of scrolling, which researchers have identified as the "dopamine loop." Dopamine is a chemical in our brains that is released after pleasure and reward-seeking behaviors—and it causes us to want them all over again. Behavioral scientist Susan Weinschenk, Ph.D., wrote:

> When you bring up the feed on one of your favorite apps, the dopamine loop has become engaged. With every photo you scroll through, headline you read, or link you go to, you are feeding the loop which just makes you want more. It takes a lot to reach satiation, and in fact, you might never be satisfied. Chances are what makes you stop is that someone interrupts you. That's why you can scroll long past the point of feeling amused or entertained by what you're seeing. You might finally close the app and think, "What did I even just read?"[2]

So just understand: **social media has a similar effect on our brains as some drugs**. We have a physical, neurological compulsion to keep logging in and scrolling. No matter the platform on which you scroll, you are likely exposed to so-called beautiful people. That has an effect on your perception of beauty whether you are aware of it at the time or not.

When you understand that, you can at least have the agency to be proactive and prevent social media from over-influencing how you perceive your own beauty.

Social Media Overexposure

Both men and women struggle with self-image issues thanks to the unrealistic beauty standards set by what they see on social media. In addition to physical issues (feeling too fat, too thin, too short, too dark, etc.), mental health issues abound as people try to achieve unattainable beauty standards.

From the minute
we open our eyes,
we are exposing
ourselves to
what is really an
alternate reality
where celebrities,
influencers, and
even friends are
trying to promote an
image of perfection
that simply exists
only online.

According to one research study, about **80% of smartphone users check their phones within fifteen minutes of waking up every morning.**[3] From the minute we open our eyes, we are exposing ourselves to what is really an alternate reality where celebrities, influencers, and even friends are trying to promote an image of perfection that simply exists only online.

In the thousands of images that appear in your feed, you see perfectly toned women with flat stomachs, long, cellulite-free legs, and perky, perfectly rounded breasts and butts. You see men with six-pack abs, bulging biceps and quads, and hairless chests. **Meanwhile, your subconscious is shaping the perfect beauty standard by which you measure yourself**. I can't stress enough—and you probably know this deep down—more often than not you are seeing a combination of intense exercise, plastic surgery, and a significant amount of filtering.

And then the likes come into play. Likes on social media allow us to signal our validation and approval with a single click. While this comes across as a fairly simple and basic feature, in reality, it is actually one of the most powerful online tools ever created. Likes first appeared on the video site Vimeo, but didn't really take off until Mark Zuckerberg and his team decided to add them to Facebook in 2009. According to digital expert Branwell Moffat, "Content on Facebook is now liked more than 3 billion times per day, and estimates suggest that since its inception, the like button has been pressed many trillions of times."[4]

Likes have become a powerful form of validation. They are the signals by which people earn approval for their physical appearance and compare themselves to others. Think about it. Have you ever felt a little disappointed when one of your posted photos gets very few likes or comments? For most of us, this is probably a minor disappointment, but for some—especially adolescents—it can cause significant anxiety.

When someone posts a "beautiful" photo of themself that garners hundreds of likes, it signals to everyone else who sees the post that this person represents a standard of beauty to which they should also aspire. In other words, we allow social media to tell us we need to be a beautiful person if we want to be worthy or "likable", which could not be further from the truth.

On top of it all, then the mental and physical health problems begin.

According to the National Eating Disorder Association, up to 70 million people around the world suffer from disordered eating (anorexia, bulimia, binge eating). Studies have clearly shown a positive correlation between the rise of social media and the rise in eating disorders, most notably among young people, but also affecting people of all ages. Why? It's easy to see that many are desperately trying to emulate the types of bodies they see receiving all of the positive attention (likes) on social media platforms.[5]

Those who don't fall into disordered eating may simply turn to the photo filters that are a part of virtually every social platform. These filters can now do anything from making you thinner (or curvier), smoothing wrinkles, hiding acne, changing facial features, whitening teeth—you name it. When compared to the dangers of eating disorders, it sounds almost harmless, right? It is, until it messes with your perception of yourself to the point that you don't want anyone to see you as anything other than your perfectly filtered self.

I know a patient personally who literally only posts filtered photos of herself. The problem is that none of the filtered photos really look like her. As a result, she's self-conscious about being in anyone else's photos because they may not filter her the way she wants to be filtered. It has become a mental health issue of sorts that she doesn't ever want to be seen online the way people see her in real life.

When filters aren't enough, real-life body modification is next. Body modification is the deliberate or permanent altering of an individual's human anatomy or appearance. In their peer-reviewed study entitled *Social Media and Its Effects on Beauty*, authors Mavis Henriques and Debasis Patnaik explain:

Body Modification involves two aspects: the processes that modify form or contours of the body such as metabolic manipulation (weight lifting, extreme dieting, use of drugs/steroids, hormones), cosmetic surgeries and procedures (liposuction, facelifts, rhinoplasty, botox, eyelash extensions), genital surgery and sex reassignment surgery, restriction or compression (waist training, foot binding), abrasion (teeth filing, scourging, flagellation), elongation (neck, lips, earlobes), partial or full removal of body parts (breasts, penis, ribs, nose, etc.), implantation of foreign objects (silicone implants, decorative items under the skin), and prosthetics (false limbs, fingernails, lenses), and processes that mark the surface of the body such as tattooing, piercing, tanning/bleaching, scarification, branding and hair removal.[6]

We have all undertaken some form of body modification by this definition; it can, however, become extreme, which is often an indicator of a mental health issue, as well. This is also why we truly need ethical plastic surgeons to look past the paycheck and say, "No. You don't need more surgery, and I'm not doing it."

The Best Defense

So how can we protect ourselves from the increasingly damaging effects of social media on self-image?

The government in Norway has taken steps to minimize the negative impact of social media by proposing a law that will require sponsored posts to label where a body's shape, size, or skin has been changed through photo manipulation or filtering. Examples include enlarged lips, exaggerated muscles, and narrowed waists. Failure to comply will result in escalating fines and **possibly even imprisonment** in extreme cases.[7]

In France, any commercial image that has been digitally altered to make a model look thinner must have a cigarette-packet style warning on it saying "photographie retouchée" or "edited photograph."[8] The Photoshop Law in Israel requires models to have a BMI of at least 18.5 BMI and for advertisers to label retouched images. In the US, the Federal Trade Commission has been enforcing truth-in-advertising laws for a hundred years, but they have been slow to respond to image retouching in advertising and social media.[9] But no one should ultimately rely on legislation to be the social media filter; it's on you to protect yourself.

If you were to get a speeding ticket and have to take a defensive driving course, you would learn tactics to help you be more aware of your surroundings at all times. It's really the same for social media. I'm not telling you not to visit these sites—they can be great tools for staying in touch with friends and family or sharing positivity in the world. But before you engage, you need a plan for your safety and sanity.

First, I would really encourage you to **manage how much time you spend on social media sites**. Make liberal use of your ability to hide or block people who make you feel worse about yourself, either directly or indirectly. Do not hesitate to block someone who comes at you with unkind comments. Seriously think about whether you should follow someone who only posts selfies that show himself or herself in an impossibly beautiful image. Generally, your best defense is simply to assume that the image of a perfectly beautiful person you are seeing is not real. So why would you let a fake image of someone else make you feel less beautiful yourself?

Remember that humans by nature are always signaling. More time is spent worrying about what people think about us than what we think about ourselves. It's time to put more awareness into reversing that ratio.

Beauty Notes

* Social media has an enormous shaping impact on our mindset. We know it profoundly impacts everyone's perceptions of beauty. It's not going anywhere, though, so the best line of defense is first to be aware of its impact.

* Both men and women struggle with self-image issues thanks to the unrealistic beauty standards set by what they see on social media. In addition to physical issues (feeling too fat, too thin, too short, too dark, etc.), mental health issues abound as people try to achieve unattainable beauty standards.

* Manage how much time you spend on social media sites. Make liberal use of your ability to hide or block people who make you feel worse about yourself, either directly or indirectly. Generally, your best defense is simply to assume that the image of a perfectly beautiful person you are seeing is not real.

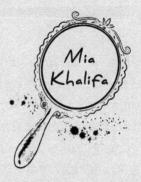

Mia
Khalifa

Mia Khalifa is a Lebanese American social media influencer with more than twenty-seven million followers on Instagram alone as of this writing. A quick look at her Instagram feed reveals a young woman with golden-brown skin, long chestnut hair with caramel highlights, and deep brown eyes. By any standard, she is absolutely beautiful.

And yet, just like every other person on the planet, she has struggled to see herself that way.

Mia was born in Beirut, Lebanon but moved to Montgomery County, Maryland when she was a very young girl. Though she spoke fluent Arabic and French, her English was limited, so she was placed in a special ESOL class in her elementary school along with some kids from Mexico and El Salvador. As a result, she often felt excluded, not just from the predominantly white and Jewish population of the school, but also from the others in her ESOL class, who excluded her because she was "the wrong kind of brown."

Feeling "ugly" because of her skin color was nothing new, though. Even in Lebanon, she was darker than many girls. The beauty standard in Beirut is more closely aligned to Western beauty standards than Middle Eastern beauty, partly because Lebanon was colonized by France. Consequently, family members would tell Mia, "Stay out of the sun; you're going to get darker...You look so much better in the winter when your skin is lighter..."

Mia picked up English quickly and was only in the ESOL program for about six months before she was moved into a regular classroom, but she had an Arabic accent for a few more years, which, along with her appearance, made her the target of bullies. In addition to having darker skin, Mia had what is often called a "unibrow" that made her look different than Caucasian girls. Desperate to get rid of it, and forbidden to have it waxed or plucked, she tried taking a razor and shaving between her brows, which didn't exactly turn out as she hoped, leaving a noticeably too-wide gap.

In the culture Mia grew up in, having a nose job or having breast implants done as a teenager is very common, and is almost a standard thing to do when you turn sixteen. Being overweight, even a little bit, is cause for disdain. It puts a lot of pressure on girls, and messes with their mental health—Mia was no exception.

She recalls, "My mental health, looking back on it, was terrible. I was constantly stressed. I had a terrible relationship with food...like if I really, really wanted something, I would feel so guilty with every single bite that I took because I felt like I was basically proving everybody right who said all of those mean things about me and about my weight.

I didn't really come into my confidence until I was twenty-three, twenty-four...I had lost weight by the time I was nineteen, and I had gotten my breast augmentation when I was twenty-one, but my mentality still hadn't caught up to the way I looked. So I still felt very, very, very self-conscious about the rest of the things that I couldn't change, like my skin tone, my eyebrows, my nose.

I just did not want to look ethnic. I wanted to look the way I was pressured to look my entire life, and I didn't start actually appreciating the fact that I look Lebanese and the fact that I don't look like everybody else until maybe two years ago, before I got my nose done.

Since then, I have come to accept and even embrace my Middle Eastern features. I love the fact that my eyebrows are thick and I never have to draw them in. And I love the fact that with this gift comes the curse of back hair and toe hair. All of these things are a package, and I wouldn't trade them for the entire world because this is all I have that connects me to my ethnicity and to my culture."

Even so, Mia is just like the rest of us and still has to filter all of the outside voices trying to make her feel less than beautiful. With millions of followers on social media, she has to ignore dozens, if not hundreds, of trolls and haters throwing shade her way every day. At one point, it was a makeup artist she hired who crossed the line:

"It was right before the Grammys, and I was very excited about going, so I spent a crazy amount of money to have my hair and makeup done. I thought I looked so beautiful. I had never felt prettier. I loved everything about the way the makeup artist did my hair and makeup.

As I was on the way to the ceremony, I got a text message from the makeup artist with a photo he had taken of me. I opened it and I was like, *What is this artificial intelligence? Who is this person?* He made my eyes bigger, my nose smaller, my lips bigger, and changed the shape of my entire jaw. I just looked like a fake, overly-airbrushed version of this person I didn't even recognize. And I got really, really upset about it!

When I opened it, my first thought was, *Wow, I suddenly feel really bad about this beautiful glam that I just had put on me. I don't even like the way I look anymore, this version of whatever person you just fabricated out of thin air.*

And what was worse was that when I showed the photo to the people around me, their reaction was, 'You look beautiful. What do you mean? Who cares if it's a little edited?' I was like, *How are you missing the point that this is not me?* I spent $3,000 to get my hair and makeup done, just for someone to throw up a basic Instagram face filter on top of it and ruin the whole thing? I had to ask him not to post it. It was a huge thing. It was awful.

I actually am actively against people who edit their photos to the extent of not being recognizable, especially if they have followings, and especially if they have young women looking up to them. Too many women want to be airbrushed beyond recognition because they can't stand to look at themselves in the mirror and appreciate their flaws and imperfections.

I have really bad days where I feel like crap and I look like crap, and I have a raging cystic acne all over my cheeks. I try to go out of my way to show that on my social posts just as much as I show when I'm glammed up and when I have my makeup done. Because that is real life. I have my makeup done three or four days a month, maybe, I don't want someone to meet me in person and think, *Oh my God, she looks nothing like she does online.*"

Mia's story really underscores how connected we all are in our self-perception of beauty, and how we all have moments of insecurity. If even this extraordinarily beautiful young woman says she has days where she feels less than attractive, why would you be any different?

The truth she understands—and you should too!—is that even on days like that, celebrity or not, you are still a beautiful person exactly as you are. Embrace it.

The War on Wrinkles

Going to great lengths to avoid the appearance of aging is nothing new. Legend has it that in 1609, Hungarian Countess Erzebet Bathory (arrested and named as a serial murderer) bathed in the blood of girls and young women to stay looking young.[1] Crazy, right?

Even more famously remembered, in 2013, Kim Kardashian underwent a "vampire facial" on her reality show. The procedure uses someone's own blood components—platelet-rich plasma—injected into and formed as a mask over the face to help them look younger. Less gruesome? Maybe.

Yet there has been a recent revival in research of using young blood drawn from teenagers and young adults and transfusing it into older adults wishing to anti-age by a process known as parabiosis. This was even parodied on Mike Judge's popular TV sitcom, *Silicon Valley*, where the antagonist tech guru, Gavin Belson (a character written based on the life of Peter Thiel, PayPal founder and early Facebook investor), in his pursuit of anti-aging has a "blood boy" following him around to donate blood at comically random moments.

Women and men alike spend billions of dollars annually on anti-aging products, including everything from skin cream to hair dye, collagen supplements to cosmetic procedures. According to one study, **the global anti-aging market was valued at over $44 billion** in 2020 and is on track for revenue of over $64 billion by 2026.[2] As a society, we are spending a lot of money to fight the inevitable signs of aging. But it's ultimately a losing battle. You are going to age. There is no way possible—surgically or otherwise—for you to look twenty-something your entire life.

You are
going to age.
There is no
way possible—
surgically or
otherwise—
for you to
look twenty-
something your
entire life.

Dr. Hanne Blank, author of *Our Bodies, Ourselves*, puts it this way:

> If you are lucky enough to live long enough your body will change. Not "might," not "could," it will change. And it may change more than once. Thankfully, this is exactly what is supposed to happen. It's literally written in your DNA. There is no wrong way to have a body. Your body is what makes you possible, and as long as it's succeeding in that job, it is an excellent body.[3]

Aging is a privilege denied to far too many people— *nearly one of every three people dies before reaching age sixty-five.* **Every single day you wake up, you are one of the lucky ones.** So why spend your days fretting about wrinkles, grey hair, age spots, or a few extra pounds?

A Losing Battle

Why do people feel so compelled to fight the appearance of aging? One primary reason is that when we look in the mirror and see ourselves looking older, we are reminded of our mortality. Death is an inevitability, but we don't like to dwell on it. And we certainly don't want to see reminders that it is coming our way.

Yes, you are going to die—hopefully after living a long, rich life full of growth and change. **So why not embrace the positives?** For example, studies have shown you're likely to be happier and less inclined to get angry as you age, likely due to the ability to control your emotions better while focusing on making the most of your life.[4] Older adults report less stress than their younger counterparts, according to the American Psychological Association's annual *Stress in America* report.[5]

Although life will always be uncertain by nature, as we move into middle age, our lives have hopefully reached a level of reasonable stability.

Another reason so many have trouble accepting aging has to do with how much your appearance defined you in your youth. If you were popular for being one of the prettiest girls in your class, or the hottest guy in school, then losing your youthful beauty may be harder to accept. It defined you, and if that's *all* that defined you, you are left with an empty identity a decade or two down the road. That's why it is even more important for the youth today to find an identity outside of looks alone.

Myth-Busting Anti-Aging Options

If you're over forty, I'll bet you've bought an anti-aging product of some sort. Some, like hair color, do what they say they'll do—yes, less grey hair does tend to look younger. (Although more and more people are going natural these days and rocking the look!) But there are countless products at every end of the price spectrum that claim to erase wrinkles, lift sagging skin, or erase age spots, that may or may not deliver what they promise. Let's look at some of the commonly-held beliefs about anti-aging options and do a little myth-busting.

Myth 1: *The more expensive, the better the anti-aging product.*

At the time of this writing, the most expensive anti-wrinkle product I could find is called JK7 Rejuvenating Serum—$1,800 for one fluid ounce. Its makers claim the benefits come from the "purest, most expensive essential oils (one of which costs up to $20,000 per liter) such as Jasmine, Rose, and Chamomile signature extracts that cost about $50,000 per liter, plus natural-based herbal liposomes, proteins, and peptides."[6] According to the company website, "it promotes healthy cell growth from below your skin's barrier, reduces wrinkle depth, and supports your skin´s vital function by building a protective layer for your skin."

That all sounds great, but remember what we discussed in Chapter Six; in all advertising, you are being sold. Aging expert and biologist Matt Kaeberlein, who is also a professor of pathology, has found that all anti-aging products, no matter the price tag, have almost nothing to do with the biological aging process. "There is no evidence to suggest that a product like this could actually impact the aging process."[7]

Myth 2: This product is scientifically proven to reduce the signs of aging.

A quick Google search reveals that just about every single product available to fight wrinkles makes a claim to be scientifically or clinically proven or backed by doctors. Remember, you are being sold. Kaeberlein explains:

> Consumers should be wary of the phrase "scientifically proven." First, if the researchers were paid by the manufacturer to do the experiment–that represents a conflict of interest which they need to declare and reduces confidence in any results they get. Second, it would be important to know whether these results have been published in a rigorous, peer-reviewed scientific journal. Third, the scientific method very rarely "proves" anything. Rigorous experimental design is aimed at disproving hypotheses, not proving them.[8]

In fact, cosmetic giant, L'Oreal got into trouble with the FTC by claiming clinically proven results with their Lancôme Génifique and L'Oréal Paris Youth Code skin care products. The claims were simply not true. L'Oreal reached a settlement with the FTC that prohibits them from making claims in advertising that their facial skin care products target or boost the activity of genes to make skin look or act younger.[9]

Myth 3: Collagen is the answer to fighting wrinkles.

New fads surface all the time when it comes to fighting the signs of aging. One of the newest is collagen. Many cosmetic brands have begun adding collagen to their creams, lotions, and serums. Yet even the most basic study of skin anatomy shows that collagen is produced in the deeper level of the skin, called the dermis (which is lower than the epidermis), so it would be difficult for collagen applied topically to actually penetrate to where it might do any good.

Knowing this, plenty of companies focus on internal consumption of collagen via supplemental powders, liquids, or pills. Some studies have shown

that ingesting collagen supplements may have beneficial effects on skin elasticity, but many of these
studies are small and funded by the companies that
make the product, increasing the opportunity for
bias in the results.[10] Additionally, collagen is a large
molecule, so absorption can be tricky. For a supple-
ment to have a chance at being effective (and only
after long-term use) it must be delivered in a smaller
peptide format which can pass more easily through
the intestinal barrier and into the bloodstream.

Myth 4: Anti-aging treatments at a doctor's office are the most effective.

While it's true that dermatologists, plastic surgeons, and some other specialists offer anti-aging
treatments you cannot access outside of their office,
even these solutions are limited in their effective-
ness. And remember—doctors profit from cosmetic
procedures, so you are still being sold! (Hopefully,
doctors do so with a level of integrity and honesty.)

Botox injections last three to four months and
cost $300 to $1,200, according to the needs of the
patient. Facial fillers last between six months and a
year and run between $600 and $1,000 per syringe.

The amount of filler used depends on the treatment area and your personal goals, but for full face management, often three or four syringes could be common in a treatment. That's no small investment to repeat indefinitely a couple of times per year.

Laser treatment for wrinkles is longer-lasting, but also more costly. Different types of lasers achieve different results, some requiring longer recovery than others. For example, the recovery time for CO_2 laser resurfacing will generally take up to two weeks, while erbium laser resurfacing usually takes one full week to recover. The cost for treatment varies depending on the type of laser and even where you live. In general, the minimum investment will be no less than $2,000. Remember: it is by no means a permanent solution. Yes, you'll experience a reduction in wrinkles, but, I hate to break it to you—you'll continue to age after the procedure which means more wrinkles.

Facelifts are the longest-lasting option for reducing wrinkles and loss of elasticity in facial skin, but even they are not permanent. As with other procedures, there are different types of facelifts. The so-called lunch-hour facelift is not a true facelift procedure, but is popular for people who have only minimal sagging. It has minimal recovery time because it only involves small cuts and sutures versus fully elevating the deeper tissues of the face in a full facelift. This mini-lift can cost between $3,500 and $8,000 and last upwards of two years.

A full facelift requires up to two weeks of recovery and will cost a minimum of $10,000 and up to $200,000. It is a more involved procedure including general anesthesia, so it is not to be taken lightly. In general, a full facelift will last approximately five to ten years before the skin begins to droop again.

Whether you're trying to fight the signs of aging by investing in a lotion or a surgical procedure, remember this: nothing is going to stop your skin from aging in the long run. You could spend tens of thousands of dollars, and, in the end, you are still going to age. So if you are interested in continued maintenance, it's ok, as products and procedures are plentiful albeit expensive. For many of us, at some point, it's time to think about growing old gracefully and embracing the beauty that comes from a life well-lived.

Men and Aging

While I recognize that women tend to be the bigger consumers of beauty products, including anti-aging products, it's important to note that men are concerned about signs of aging, too. One of the biggest concerns men have around aging is with their hair—specifically, hair loss.

You may hear a good-looking older man referred to as a "silver fox", meaning he has mostly grey or white hair. So, in many ways, it's not the loss of color that is of the biggest concern. If you're a silver fox, you at least have hair! **It's *not* having hair that men tend to dread**. For some, the loss of hair signals a loss of control in their lives. They often have increased anxiety and despair due to an inability to stop their changing appearance.

"For men in our culture, in general, hair is associated with masculinity and virility and being a 'real man,'" says Gershen Kaufman, Ph.D. And when a man is "faced with the awareness that I am not what I used to be, that's infused with shame."[11]

In the United States alone, men spend nearly $4 billion annually on hair loss prevention and restoration products including medications, shampoos, even surgical measures, to save their strands. Just as with cosmetic products marketed to women, these products often make claims that aren't totally accurate. In just one example, the FTC cracked down on a company called Nutriol for claims that its products would "stop, prevent, cure, relieve, reverse, or reduce hair loss and promote the growth of hair where hair has already been lost"[12]

It's safe to say hair loss is the number one concern men have around aging, more than wrinkles, or weight gain, or anything else that might make them seem less attractive. **What's interesting is that women really don't notice or mind men with less hair.** In fact, a recent study revealed that fully 97% of women are unaffected by "minor hair loss" on a guy. And 76% of women say they would even date a guy with "severe" hair loss. This reality simply highlights the fact that sometimes what bothers us most when we look in the mirror isn't even noticed when we go out in the world!

Words of Encouragement

I live in Los Angeles, so obviously I'm in an environment where celebrities who make their living in
television or movies spend hundreds of thousands
of dollars to maintain a youthful appearance. I am
a big believer that if you feel more beautiful about
yourself when you've had a little work done, great!
Go for it! But we've all seen what it looks like when a
woman gets one too many facelifts or has had a little
too much botox or lip plumper. **There is definitely
a line you really don't want to cross.**

I think it's so encouraging when women who are in the spotlight age more naturally (with minimal or no surgical intervention) and embrace the beauty that comes with age. And they aren't afraid to speak out about it:

"We live in a youth-obsessed culture that is constantly trying to tell us that if we are not young, and we're not glowing, and we're not hot, that we don't matter. I refuse to let a system or a culture or a distorted view of reality tell me that I don't matter. I know that only by owning who and what you are can you start to step into the fullness of life. Every year should be teaching us all something valuable. Whether you get the lesson is really up to you."

–Oprah Winfrey

"If I wanted to be prettier, fillers, Botox and a neck lift might help – but I think I'm past all that. My feelings come out in my face and show who I am inside in ways that words can't express. In fact, I'm confused by what 'authentic' is; am I less authentic because I wear 'eccentric' clothes and hats? No. I look at my contemporaries who have had 'good work' done; are they less authentic? No! And neither are the women who've had procedures that went awry."

–Diane Keaton

"There is a saying that with age, you look outside what you are inside. If you are someone who never smiles your face gets saggy. If you're a person who smiles a lot, you will have more smile lines. Your wrinkles reflect the roads you have taken; they form the map of your life."

–Diane Von Furstenburg

> "In interviews, the first question I get in America is always: 'What do you do to stay young?' I do nothing. I don't think aging is a problem...Yes, my face has wrinkles. But I don't find it monstrous. I'm so surprised that the emphasis on aging here is on physical decay, when aging brings such incredible freedom."
>
> —Isabella Rossellini

So many young girls today use filters on their Snapchat or other social posts to look older than they are—a potentially dangerous habit that could take up a whole chapter on its own. It's really disturbing to see a twelve-year-old girl come off as a twenty-three-year-old woman. Meanwhile, more mature women are using those same filters to look younger, magically erasing any signs of aging. You'd think the twenty-somethings would be happy since everyone is trying to filter to look like them, but they're using filters, too!

When you realize that almost everyone thinks the grass is greener when you're younger or when you're older, depending on which side of the fence you're on, **it kind of makes all of the worry spent on the aging issue seem pointless,** doesn't it?

I encourage you to take some time right now to really appreciate your age, whatever it is. Think of all of the things that you wouldn't have experienced if you hadn't been blessed to live as long as you have. Think of all of the things you'll miss if you don't get to live to have double or triple the wrinkles and grey hair you do today.

Aging is the greatest privilege of all, and I encourage you to recognize that, embrace it, and then look in the mirror and be grateful for the reflection.

Beauty Notes

* As a society, we are spending a lot of money to fight the inevitable signs of aging. But it's ultimately a losing battle. You are going to age. There is no way possible—surgically or otherwise—for you to look twenty-something your entire life.

* Aging is a privilege denied to far too many people—nearly one of every three people dies before reaching age sixty-five. Every single day you wake up, you are one of the lucky ones. So why spend your days fretting about wrinkles, grey hair, age spots, or a few extra pounds?

* Whether you're trying to fight the signs of aging by investing in a lotion or a surgical procedure, remember this: nothing is going to stop your skin from aging in the long run. You could spend tens of thousands of dollars, and, in the end, you are still going to age. It's time to think about growing old gracefully and embracing the beauty that comes from a life well-lived.

9

See Yourself As You Really Are

———

Alice Walker is an African American novelist, poet, and essayist. She is the first African American woman to have won the Pulitzer Prize for fiction. In her essay, "Beauty: When the Other Dancer Is the Self," she shares her own struggle with self-image and her journey to accepting her true beauty.[1]

When she was young, she was identified as the "pretty little girl" who loved to dress up in her crinoline dress, polished patent-leather shoes, and colorful hair ribbons. At age two-and-a-half, she entreated her father to choose her from among her siblings to accompany him to the county fair declaring, "I'm the prettiest!"

At age six, after standing in front of her church congregation and flawlessly reciting an Easter speech, she basked in the praise, "Oh, isn't she the *cutest* thing!"

Two years later, everything changed. While playing cowboys and Indians with her brothers and their BB guns in their backyard one day, she was suddenly and accidentally shot with a BB in her right eye. Her brothers, scared of getting in deep trouble, convinced her to not tell her parents the truth about what happened. Instead, they told her to say she tripped over a piece of wire that flew up and hit her in the eye.

One week later, with her injury becoming infected and getting much worse, she finally admitted what had really happened and was taken to see a doctor. At that point, there was no chance of saving her eye. But worse than the blindness, Alice was upset by the glob of white-colored scar tissue that remained on her eye.

She writes, "Now when I stare at people—a favorite pastime, up to now—they will stare back. Not at the 'cute' little girl, but at her scar. For six years I do not stare at anyone, because I do not raise my head."

She did everything she could to avoid having people look at her, but still she was teased and bullied by schoolmates. She would hide in her room when relatives came to visit. She writes that every night she would look in the mirror and "rant and rave at it... plead with it to clear up...tell it I hate and despise it. I do not pray for sight. I pray for beauty."

At age fourteen she was visiting an older brother in Boston who understood her feelings of ugliness and took her to a doctor. This specialist was able to remove the scar tissue, but a small blue crater was left in its place. For Alice, this was preferable to the ugly white blob, so she felt somewhat better, but still not beautiful.

It wasn't until she was twenty-seven that Alice's three-year-old daughter suddenly noticed the blue mark in her mother's eye. Alice writes:

> She studies my face intently…she even holds my face maternally between her dimpled little hands. Then, looking every bit as serious and lawyerlike as her father, she says, as if it may just possibly have slipped my attention: "Mommy, there's a world in your eye…where did you get that world in your eye."

In that moment, Alice realized that it was possible to love that world in her eye. The sweet innocence of a child's awe-filled observation changed her perspective.

Alice concludes her moving essay by sharing a dream she had that same night, in which she was happily dancing and whirling around and was joined by another dancer, her other self: "She is beautiful, whole, and free. And she is also me."

Be-YOU-tiful as You Are

The person you are today is incredible. You have so many unique, wonderful qualities that it would be nearly impossible to list them all. You don't have to be a certain size or shape; you don't have to have a certain skin, hair, or eye color. No matter your age, you have a body with strengths and weaknesses, features and flaws. Being alive in that body—just exactly as it is today—is a gift. **It's time to start viewing it as such.**

If you are having trouble accepting the truth of your beauty, you need to work on your mindset. Even a small shift in mindset can help you to see yourself in a whole new light. Right now, you may think that in order to feel attractive, desirable—yes, beautiful!—your outward appearance has to align with all of the artificial beauty standards I exposed in previous chapters.

In fact, there are simple lifestyle adjustments—mental and physical—you can make that have been shown in numerous studies to help you feel more satisfied with your body and appearance.[2] **In other words, you can choose to see yourself as beautiful**.

🐮 Clear Your Mind.

> Before you can add any of the following
> practices to your life, you have to clear
> mental space for them to be effective.
> If your mind is full of negative thoughts
> about yourself, there is no room for the
> good to come in and effect change.

Let me demonstrate. Right now, take a deep breath
and hold it for as long as you can. (Really, go ahead!
I'll wait.) When you can't hold it any longer, when
you need more air, go ahead and stop holding.

What is the first thing you did? Was it to suck in
more air? No, you exhaled first. By exhaling, you
cleared your lungs of carbon dioxide, a toxic waste
gas, before you breathed in new, clean oxygen.

It works the same way with your mind. You have to
empty it of all of your toxic thoughts, beliefs, and
paradigms before you bring in the newer, healthier,
more freeing thoughts and perceptions.

One of the
best ways I
know to change
your mindset,
clear out the
negative, and
make way for
the positive is
by practicing
gratitude.

One of the best ways I know to change your mindset, clear out the negative, and make way for the positive is by practicing gratitude. Take a few minutes each day, ideally at the beginning of the day, to think of at least three things you are grateful for. Of course, you can acknowledge the big things: your health, your family, clean water, abundant food, and so on. But I also encourage you to find the small things to be grateful for: your steaming mug of coffee, a text from a friend, sunshine, your baby's giggle.

Many people find that keeping these thoughts in a gratitude journal is a great way to challenge yourself to come up with new things to be grateful for each day. Reading back over what you wrote is always a mood booster when you start to feel that negative mental mindset creeping back in.

If you really struggle to overcome negative thinking and find things to be grateful for in your life, I recommend seeking help from a therapist or counselor. A mental health professional may provide a fresh perspective and help you have a better understanding of your thoughts and emotions so that you can flip the script and begin to see things in a healthier, more positive way.

When you are able to eliminate your toxic thoughts about yourself and become open to seeing yourself as the beautiful person you are, you can begin to take more of the following steps.

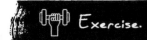 Exercise.

Obviously, exercise can have a physical effect on your appearance, and I don't just mean making you thinner or more toned. When you move your body regularly, oxygen is pumped through the blood and you experience improved circulation, even at rest. Your body's cells—including skin cells—are nourished by the increased blood flow which leads to more effective cellular repair and replacement. In other words, your skin cells are healthier, which will give you that so-called healthy glow.

Beyond that, studies have shown that moderate exercise can help prevent and reverse the signs of aging. A research study including individuals six-ty-five and older who exercised more frequently had healthy skin resembling individuals of much younger ages. With just thirty minutes of moderate exercise each day, it is possible for you to turn back the clock for your skin.

Exercise also increases confidence, and confident people tend to radiate physical appeal and charisma. The effects of exercise on self-worth happen even before measurable physical changes related to exercise are observed, which means once you start moving your body, your energy levels go up. That is directly tied to your self-assurance. Nothing is more beautiful than feeling good in your own skin.

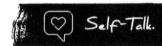

♡ Self-Talk.

It seems logical that getting praise and compliments from others would be the best way to boost your self-image. In actuality, neuroscience studies have shown that your inner voice, the way you "speak" to yourself, is far more powerful.[3]

During a moment of frustration, have you ever spoken rudely to someone? *Watch how you speak to me!* may be the response you heard, and afterwards, you probably regretted your words to some degree. We have all been programmed to be careful of how we speak to others because we know how powerful our words can be. As a result, we are conscious of how we speak to our parents, grandparents, bosses, employees, loved ones, strangers, waiters, janitors—everyone except ourselves!

With ourselves, we often forget how powerful our words can be, and the harmful repercussions negative self-language can have. It may feel a little awkward, but repeating positive affirmations to yourself in the mirror, or saying things that you like about yourself will help you validate those traits and value them in yourself.

But first, right now, before we go any further, I want you to look in the mirror and tell the person looking back loudly and clearly: "Watch how you speak to me!"

Now we can continue!

I'm not really a fan of the pre-packaged one-size-fits-all affirmations that you can find with a quick Google search: *I am kind. I am worthy. I am smart.* I believe it is far more useful to write and then say affirmations you come up with that are unique and purposeful.

Start by being honest about the negative things you are telling yourself. *I can't lose weight. I'm not smart enough for that job. I have too many wrinkles.* Whatever it is, write it down. Then flip the script. Imagine the world was perfect, and rewrite those negatives as positives. *I am capable of becoming fit and healthy. I am smart and learn more every day. I have been blessed to grow older and have beautiful smile lines to show for it.*

Going forward, whenever you catch yourself having negative thoughts or feelings about yourself, flip the script. Don't feed the negativity; rather, shine some light on it and reframe it in a way that will boost your self-assurance.

Then, every morning when you look at yourself in the mirror, be your own hype squad. Speak aloud your positive affirmations. And if you want to take it a step further, try doing what Mel Robbins, author of *The High 5 Habit*, does—give yourself a high five in the mirror!

Smile and Laugh—Often.

While you're looking in the mirror and reciting affirmations, try smiling. It's no surprise that smiling makes you seem warm, attractive, and approachable to others, but you can get the same benefits from smiling in the mirror. Research has shown that you receive similar neural cues when you see yourself smile as if a familiar friend smiles at you.[4]

Laughing can help you see yourself in a more positive light. When someone takes themself and every aspect of their life too seriously, it shows on their face. Being able to laugh off the small things that might get under your skin will make you more relaxed, which in turn will be reflected in a more pleasant appearance.

A study by the University of Kansas found that laughing with another person can increase attraction, too. In the study, pairs of people who didn't know each other talked, and the more the pair laughed together, the higher level of attraction they reported.[5]

🌟 💬 Boost Your Confidence.

Confidence comes across the minute you enter a room. It's in your smile, your body language, and your eye contact. When you are feeling awkward, people pick up on that, and it can affect how they perceive you.

Having good posture can make you look good, but it can also make you feel good.

A study from the Association of Psychological Science found that just sitting up straight can make you feel more confident and powerful.[6] So the saying "keep your chin up" can be taken literally as well as figuratively when you're looking for a confidence boost.

Choose to dress in a way that you can feel comfortable and confident. This means you choose clothes that fit well and flatter you, no matter your size or shape. Love color? Go for it! You'll feel far more confident rocking a color or pattern you love than if you try to virtually disappear by wearing muted neutrals. Of course, if black or neutrals are your jam, and you feel gorgeous wearing them, then you do you!

If you feel better about yourself when you're wearing a little makeup, or have some Botox or other cosmetic treatments, then, by all means, go for it! Every day I see how people can feel more confident, and therefore more beautiful, by enhancing their appearance artificially, and that's fine. When you choose that bright red lipstick because it makes you feel gorgeous, and not because an advertisement made you think you needed to have it, you're empowered.

In the same way, you shouldn't feel like you have to be made-up to feel like your most gorgeous self. If your all-natural, makeup-free look is how you feel best about yourself, you're also empowered! When you're empowered, you're confident. And confidence is beautiful.

😊😊 Examine Your Friendships.

In Chapter 8, we looked at how to edit your online friendships and be intentional about whose posts you follow. The same principle applies to your real-life friendships. Allowing a toxic person to be part of your life may be preventing you from feeling your best.

If you have so-called friends who are constantly negative, put people down, act or speak rudely, or make little jokes—even about you, sometimes!—it's time to cut those people out of your life or spend significantly less time with them.

Or maybe you have friends who don't do any of those obviously toxic things, but they constantly fixate on their own appearance: *Does this make me look fat? Oh, I'm having such a bad hair day. Ugh, I can't deal with this breakout!* You can't spend time around someone who obsesses about their appearance without starting to adopt some of the same habits. There is truth to the adage that you are much like the five people you spend the most time with.

When you choose to prioritize the people who spend their time supporting you and building you up, people who have a healthy self-image, you're naturally going to feel free to be genuinely *you*—and that is beautiful, too.

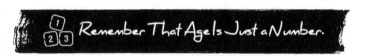

Remember That Age Is Just a Number.

The number of birthdays you've had does not have to define you. Be grateful for every single one you have, and remember that a particular number has little to do with how old you feel and look.

You get to define what it means to be attractive whether you're twenty, thirty, forty, fifty, or beyond. Find women or men in your everyday life—not "Real Housewives" or other celebrities—that you see as attractive. Let them serve as your role models for aging beautifully.

Cybill Shepherd, a beauty icon who is now in her 70s, told Oprah Winfrey in an interview that she only began to feel truly beautiful as she got older and her identity shifted away from her appearance.[7]

If you measure your beauty and your identity by the artificial beauty standard, you will find yourself struggling when you age past what that beauty standard defines as ideal.

Alice Hart-Davis, award-winning beauty journalist and author, when asked about aging, wisely said, "Now in our mid-50s, we know who we are and where we're at, more or less. We know the clothes that suit us, we know the value of hair dye and a good blow-dry and we know that lipstick, mascara, and brow pencils are our friends."[8]

So as you grow older, embrace the changes that come as part of the package. They are there to remind you of the life you've lived to this point—all of the ups and downs, easier times and harder times, joy and pain. When you can take that perspective, it frees you to appreciate who you are today.

How to Know You're Beautiful

It's no secret that we are our own harshest critics. Even in light of everything I've shared above, you may still find that the voice in your head refuses to acknowledge the myriad ways in which you are already beautiful. If that's the case, maybe you should include some trusted outside opinions.

Think about a few people that you truly love or care about, people you trust who you know will be honest with you. Step outside of your comfort zone (and ego) and ask them to tell you honestly what they find beautiful about you. Not, "Am I beautiful to you?" but "What do you find beautiful about me?"

You may ask the question hoping that they'll mention certain features you work so hard to bring to a certain standard of beauty, but I bet you'll be surprised at what you actually hear. Honestly, even as a plastic surgeon who specializes in rhinoplasty, I can say there are very few people who would name your nose as one of your most beautiful features. The reality is, people see you as a whole, not as the sum of your parts, as you are likely to see yourself when you're critiquing yourself in the mirror.

The reality
is, people see
you as a whole,
not as the
sum of your
parts, as you
are likely to see
yourself when
you're critiquing
yourself in
the mirror.

While you're busy looking for things not to love, your family and friends see your beauty and don't even think twice about any potential flaws. In fact, they probably won't even name only physical attributes when describing your beauty. Maybe you have a great, big, hearty laugh. Maybe you are empathetic and caring. Maybe you're a brilliant musician. Or an intellectual giant. **Be prepared to hear a wide range of descriptors of what's beautiful about you**, very few of which will actually be aligned with the traditional beauty standard. I know it sounds like something your mom would say, but there is so much truth to it: *your personality is largely what makes you beautiful.*

Mirrors reflect an image that tells us only on the surface what we look like. Next time you're in front of a mirror, really look at yourself, but look past your reflection, and take in who you *actually are* as a person.

What you see in the mirror is only the image that informs the world of your physical self. You know that who you are is far more than what the world sees. You have the ability to change the internal lens through which you perceive yourself. When you take back the power to define what is beautiful for you, and see yourself as you truly are, you will inevitably become more attractive to yourself and others.

We would all agree that some of the loveliest women in the world are not flawless. But they feel beautiful thanks to their confidence and their ability to enjoy life.

It's time for you to see yourself as you truly are, and do the same for others.

Beauty Notes

---

* The person you are today is incredible. You have so many unique, wonderful qualities that it would be nearly impossible to list them all. You don't have to be a certain size or shape; you don't have to have a certain skin, hair, or eye color. No matter your age, you have a body with strengths and weaknesses, features and flaws. Being alive in that body–just exactly as it is today–is a gift. It's time to start viewing it as such.

* Simple lifestyle adjustments– mental and physical–you can make that have been shown in numerous studies to help you feel more satisfied with your body and appearance include:

- Clear Your Mind
- Exercise
- Positive Self-Talk
- Smile and Laugh—Often
- Boost Your Confidence
- Examine Your Friendships
- Remember Age Is
  Just a Number

✱ What you see in the mirror is only
the image that informs the world
of your physical self. You know that
who you are is far more than what
the world sees. You have the ability
to change the internal lens through
which you perceive yourself.
When you take back the power to
define what is beautiful for you,
and see yourself as you truly are,
you will inevitably become more
attractive to yourself and others.

10

Filtering the Voices

Lizzie Velasquez was born in 1989 with a rare disease called neonatal progeria syndrome. As a result, she is blind in one eye, her craniofacial features are distorted, and the aortic valve in her heart could rupture at any time. When she was born, doctors warned her parents she would never be able to gain weight and likely never walk or talk. They brought her home, loved her, and reared her to walk and talk like any other child. It wasn't until her first day of Kindergarten that she knew there was anything different about her.

As she walked into her classroom—wearing a backpack nearly bigger than she was—she approached another little girl and smiled at her. As Lizzie describes it, "She looked up at me like I was a monster, like I was the scariest thing she had ever seen in her life. My first reaction was, *She is really rude!*... Unfortunately, the day got worse and worse. A lot of people just wanted to have nothing to do with me, and I didn't understand why. In my mind, I was a really cool kid."[1]

Lizzie went home and asked her parents what was wrong with her and why the other kids were being so mean to her. They told her that the only thing different about her was that she was smaller than the other kids, saying, "Go to school, pick your head up, smile, and continue to be yourself." She did, but the bullying never stopped.

> For so long I thought what defined me
> was my outer appearance. I thought
> that my little tiny legs, and my little
> arms, and my little face were ugly. I
> thought I was disgusting. I hated when
> I'd wake up in the morning when I was
> going to middle school, and would be
> looking in the mirror getting ready,
> and thinking, Can I just scrub this syn-
> drome off? I would wish, and pray,
> and hope, and do whatever I could so
> I would wake up in the morning and be
> different, and I wouldn't have to deal
> with these struggles. It's what I wanted
> every single day, and every single day
> I was disappointed.[2]

When she was in high school, just seventeen years old, Lizzie came across a YouTube video that someone had posted of her calling her "the world's ugliest woman." The eight-second, soundless video clip went viral with over four million views. Lizzie sat there and scrolled through thousands of hateful comments, desperate to find one person who would stand up for her. She never found it. Instead, she found, "Lizzie, please - please - just do the world a favor, put a gun to your head, and kill yourself."

It didn't take long, though, for Lizzie to realize she had a choice:

> *Am I going to let the people who called me a monster define me? Am I going to let the people who said, "Kill it with fire!" define me? No; I'm going to let my goals, and my success, and my accomplishments be the things that define me. Not my outer appearance, not the fact that I'm visually impaired, not the fact that I have this syndrome that nobody knows what it is.*[3]

Lizzie saw the supermodels on the magazine covers and the gorgeous actresses in movies and on TV and said that her idea of what beauty was "sort of just diminished; it wasn't even a thing, because if I'm the ugliest person in the world, where does that standard of beauty even begin?"[4] Instead, she made the decision to embrace gratitude.

Rather than dwell on her one blind eye, she is grateful for vision in the other eye. Instead of being upset about her tiny stature and having to buy kid-sized clothes and shoes, she is grateful she doesn't have to pay adult-sized prices. She loves and is grateful for her pretty, long, thick chestnut hair.

In an interview on the YouTube show *Pretty Unfiltered*, Lizzie was asked what beauty means to her:

> Beauty to me doesn't really mean one thing; I don't really believe that there is a set definition for all of us. I think beauty is what you decide it is. Beauty is your values, and your personality, and your goals in life, and the way you treat other people.

We can do so many things to cover up who we really are. We could dye our hair. We could put all this makeup on. We could get all these clothes. And with social media apply ten filters. You can do all of these things during the day, and you want that instant gratification of "Ok, well they liked it, so great—they're seeing this outer shell of me." But when you take all that off, if you are able to lay down at night with only who you are, if you're proud enough to carry that out the front door the next morning, that's when you know you've found what beauty is.[5]

Protective Filtering

It is unlikely you have had to endure a viral video with thousands of comments criticizing your appearance. On the flip side, you've more than likely heard or seen *something* that made you feel bad about yourself, somehow less than beautiful.

Maybe your mom made an offhand comment about a dress being too tight on you, or your sibling teased you about a bad haircut. Maybe you picked up the latest copy of *People* magazine and saw an actress who delivered a baby a month ago flaunting a belly that looked like it was never pregnant. (Apparently, doubling up on Spanx *is* a thing.)

No matter the source, something has made its way into your consciousness that negatively impacted your ability to see yourself as you truly are: *beautiful*. **I hate to break it to you, but those sources are never going away.** Not your mom. Not your sibling. Not the magazines and not the media. Anything and everything that has the ability to affect your self-image—positively or negatively—will continue to exist indefinitely.

Anything and
everything that
has the ability
to affect your
self-image—
positively or
negatively—
will continue
to exist
indefinitely.

Now for the good news: you have complete agency to minimize or eliminate the impact those negative inputs can have on you, your self-image, and your self-confidence. You are not a magnet for every negative word or thought; **you can learn to filter those voices and intentionally weed out anything that does not serve you well.**

Psychologist Dr. Nichole Wood-Barcalow and her research team coined the term "protective filtering" to describe how people—especially women— use their "protective filter to process and respond to information, typically in a self- and body-preserving manner...(they) accept information that is consistent with positive body image while rejecting messages that could endanger it."[6]

Participants in her study were female American college students, ages 18 to 25. They were exposed to an Instagram feed created specifically for the study which featured images posted by eight popular female influencers with two million or more followers who were known for their idealized physical appearance. (Think Kendall Jenner, Gigi Hadid, Michelle Lewin, etc.) The images curated for the feed emphasized appearance, exercise, food and nutrition, lifestyle, and entertainment and were deemed reflective of the current general beauty standards for women.

For the study, participants were seated in front of a laptop for ten minutes with the Instagram feed open, given a paper and pen, and instructed to write down everything that crossed their minds while viewing the images in the feed. Following this ten-minute period, each participant was interviewed by a researcher for approximately an hour to record their thoughts.

What researchers observed resulted in the idea of protective filtering. For example, when participants questioned *why* the influencer was sharing a particular image, and perceived that its intent was to market or advertise something (weight loss product, makeup, brand of clothing), their protective filter kicked in and the images lost the potential to harm the participants' body image.

When participants were critical about the time and energy that these influencers likely devote to diet and exercise in order to maintain the supposedly ideal figure, and determined that to put forth such effort would interfere with activities they personally enjoyed, their protective filter kicked in again. One participant, Stefanie, suggested, "Sometimes I know that I don't look like a model and that I have more weight than the average model, but I know that I like my life as it is and I love food. I love going to restaurants with friends and family. I really don't want to exchange that for going to the gym twice a day and running five hours, not eating, or only eating vegetables, and always being so focused on my body."[7]

Almost all of the participants noted the fact that the ideal beauty standard was unrealistic for most people without cosmetic surgery or at least heavy filtering of images. When the protective filter kicked in, they focused on the fact that they virtually never encounter "idealized" bodies in their daily lives. **Rather, they are surrounded by people of all sizes, shapes, and skin colors**. One participant, Anouk, said, "It [beauty-ideal imagery] doesn't reflect our society and how women are. It doesn't represent what you see normally."

When you are aware and critical of the unrealistic requirements for meeting the traditional beauty standards, you can choose to block any imagery or messaging that might harm your positive body image. Knowing the images are not typical, and in many cases are not natural or real, you can dismiss them and move on. As Wood-Baraclow's study concluded:

> Women are confronted with potential influences on an ongoing basis, and they must, in turn, decide whether to accept or reject information...other people and negative images or messages don't control your own body image. You decide things. When it comes down to it, you make your own body image. Despite women's active commitment to protective filtering, it is not foolproof. Sometimes negative information would impact the women's positive body image, but they chose to cognitively redirect their filter to reframe the information in a neutral or positive manner so it would not impact their body image long-term.

Next time you're scrolling through your social media feed or thumbing through a fashion magazine, let your protective filter do its job. You can appreciate the beauty you see, but use the strategies mentioned above to remind yourself that what you're seeing is manipulated in some way and not necessarily portraying reality.

Negative Friends or Family

Limiting and filtering your exposure to media that leaves you feeling less is one thing. But what if some of the people in your life are those negative voices? Lizzie Velasquez grew up surrounded by a family who spoke positivity to her and encouraged her to look beyond the surface to find her true beauty. Unfortunately, that is not everyone's experience growing up.

One blogger on a parenting site shared an experience she had with her mother:

> *My mother has commented on my looks hundreds of times since I was a child, and I thought it would stop when I grew up. It hasn't. I get praise when I meet her definition of what's attractive and criticism when I don't. She said it again, just in case I hadn't heard it the first time. "Oh, now you have a pooch in the back AND in the front."*
>
> *Nobody laughed. Nothing effectively curbs her commentary, but I tried a different tack anyway: "You know what they'd call that at (my daughter's) elementary school? They'd say that was unkind."[8]*

Parents can be one of the most painful sources of negative input, yet often don't realize their words are hurtful because they are well-intentioned. If this is an issue that resonates with you, it is time to establish healthy boundaries. But how do you politely tell a parent to rein in comments that are hurtful to you?

Parents can
be one of the
most painful
sources of
negative input,
yet often don't
realize their
words are
hurtful because
they are
well-intentioned.

Therapists suggest you be specific about what you would like and what the consequences will be if the boundary is crossed. Perhaps you can say something like, "Mom, your comments about my weight are hurtful. If you comment on my weight in any way, I am not going to continue this conversation." You can expect people to have a negative reaction at first to your newly-established boundaries, but if you are determined and consistent with enforcing them, most people will eventually adjust.

In the case of the blogger above, she decided to confront her mother by writing her a letter:

It stops here. I mean that in the most respectful way... If you had lobbed your hatred of my weight at me during a time when my daughter wasn't there, it would have had a different impact. But here's something for you to think about. Is this really what you want the next generation of our family's women to learn? That it's okay to cut down a female family member based on her appearance? Is this what you want to perpetuate? ... I've learned that I am more than how I look. I accept myself. I have something to offer the world, and it can't be captured by numbers on the bathroom scale or the tags on my clothing.[9]

Remember, just because someone has said something derogatory or insensitive about your appearance, it doesn't make it true. Their words do not have the power to affect you unless you decide to take them to heart. Ask yourself if that person's opinion really matters, then make the intentional decision to let their thoughtless comments go.

Managing Input from Outsiders

We live in a day and age where the anonymity of the metaverse allows people to make comments without any ramifications. Though it is less common, sometimes people do say hurtful things to others even in real life. If someone is thoughtless, rude, or unkind, it is understandably tempting to respond angrily, but that can leave you feeling bad, too.

Instead, try some of the following tactics to let the other person know you heard them but you are not going to let their comments phase you.

* **Walk away.** If the person's comment seems to be a direct confrontation, your best bet is to just walk away, especially if you feel threatened.

Anyone who is rude enough to make negative comments about your appearance isn't going to be interested in anything you have to say back to them. When you walk away, you show that you are in control, not bothering to respond to their rudeness because they are not worth your time.

✳ **Give the person a look.** Don't say anything; just look them in the eye for a couple of seconds, then look away. You could also maintain eye contact and frown or raise your eyebrows. They will get the message.

✳ **Speak up. Be direct. But with Low Expectations.** Say something like, "I don't think it is very nice to say things about someone's appearance," or, "It seems like you have a problem with the way I look. I don't have a problem with my appearance."

✳ **Remember your positive affirmations.** If you don't feel like you can actively let someone know they are out of line, then remind *yourself* that they are wrong: *What they think is not my problem. I would never be unkind enough to speak that way. There is much more to me than one person's opinion of how I look.*

Keep the Attitude of Gratitude

The same study noted earlier in this chapter that generated the concept of protective filtering also put the spotlight on the importance of focusing gratefully on what you love and appreciate about yourself, not just in appearance, but in your body's functionality.

Over half of the participants in the study shared that rather than comparing their appearance to the women on the Instagram feed, they would focus on and express gratitude for their ability to walk, ride a bike, reach for something on a high shelf, and so on. One participant, Noa, said, "When I look at myself, I think 'oh, this is not perfect', but if that's the only thing, it's nothing compared to the things my body is capable of doing...I continue to look at how my body is perfect because it does everything I want...it just doesn't make sense to feel bad about myself because I'm really lucky to have a well-functioning body."[10]

Writing a list of what you appreciate about your body is a great way to bring your focus to what is important. Use the format of "I appreciate my [body aspect] because...." For example, you could say, "I appreciate my strong, muscular legs because they carry me wherever I have to go and allow me to continually build strength in my yoga practice."[11] Maybe you appreciate your face because it reminds you of your mom. Or you appreciate your strong, healthy teeth because they let you enjoy steak dinners! Let yourself be free and creative as you think about the myriad ways you love so many things about your body.

No matter what you see in the mirror, it's up to you to decide to be comfortable in your own skin. That can be a challenge in a society that values unrealistic images, but it is possible to filter the inputs you receive and retrain your brain on how to think positively about your reflection and your body. Telling yourself that you're beautiful, even when it feels hard to believe at first, will eventually build your confidence. And nothing is more beautiful than a confident person, comfortable in their own skin.

Note: If negative thoughts about your body become overwhelming and you find it hard to give up perfectionistic habits about food, weight, or exercise, consult your doctor, therapist, or a counselor.

Beauty Notes

* *No matter the source, something has
  made its way into your consciousness
  that negatively impacted your ability
  to see yourself as you truly are:
  beautiful. Those sources are never
  going away. Anything and everything
  that has the ability to affect your
  self-image—positively or negatively—
  will continue to exist indefinitely.*

* *Now for the good news: you have
  complete agency to minimize or
  eliminate the impact those negative
  inputs can have on you, your self-
  image, and your self-confidence.
  You are not a magnet for every
  negative word or thought; you can
  learn to filter those voices and
  intentionally weed out anything
  that does not serve you well.*

* When you are aware and critical of the unrealistic requirements for meeting the traditional beauty standards, you can choose to block any imagery or messaging that might harm your positive body image. Knowing the images are not typical, and in many cases are not natural or real, you can dismiss them and move on.

* Remember, just because someone has said something derogatory or insensitive about your appearance, it doesn't make it true. Their words do not have the power to affect you unless you decide to take them to heart. Ask yourself if that person's opinion really matters, then make the intentional decision to let their thoughtless comments go.

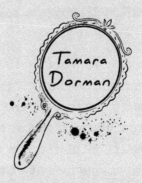

Tamara Dorman is a Southern California native, co-founder of BĀBEN swimwear, and successful real estate agent in the luxury home market. She's a beautiful woman who naturally falls in line with the beauty ideal of the blonde, tan, gorgeous "California girl."

And just like everyone else, she has dealt with insecurity about her appearance.

When she was just seventeen years old, she had a boyfriend who became physically abusive, something she hid from her single mom and her older brother who was in college. As with many victims of domestic abuse, she felt somehow embarrassed and unsure of what to do about it, so she covered for him.

On one occasion, he hit her so hard in her nose that she was pretty sure he broke it. She ended up with black eyes that she hid from her mom by staying at his house and telling her she'd been in a car accident and hit the dashboard.

She says, "I probably should have gone to a doctor when it happened, and maybe they would have done something at that point to straighten it out. But I was afraid of him, and still stayed with him. I was young and insecure."

Eventually (thankfully!) she broke up with him, went off to college, and pushed that dark time out of her mind. She went on to marry and have twins—a boy and a girl—who have grown up to be successful young adults.

Several years ago, a couple of decades after this happened, Tamara started noticing her nose in photos, thinking it looked a little crooked and maybe wider on the bridge than it was when she was young. She knew that it was probably because of that traumatic punch in the face from when she was younger, and the upsetting memories rose to the surface again.

The more she dwelled on her nose, the bigger the problem seemed, and the more she wanted to get rid of it—the bump AND the memory. That's when she came to see me for a consultation.

Tamara recalls, "I went in for the visit, had some pictures taken, and was expecting to make an appointment to have the surgery. Dr. Dugar said, 'Can I be honest with you? You don't need to do anything with your nose. If I did something, first of all, it's going to cost a lot of money. And it's so slight that you may end up looking worse.' I'm really kind of thankful he said that. It changed my perspective. I realized that the memory I was trying to suppress was giving me a distorted perception of how my nose actually looks. After that conversation, I've put it out of my mind, and I haven't really thought about it since!"

BĀBEN, the swimwear company Tamara co-founded with her fashion-designer daughter Hanna, states its mission is "to empower and to connect to all women, and to be with them on their way to learning to love and adorn their bodies."

Tamara reflects, "It's about just appreciating all beauty, all sizes, and all kinds of faces. It's interesting how you can appreciate the beauty in so many other people, and things they find fault with you would never even notice. But when it comes to yourself, somehow you can be a little more unappreciative or ungrateful."

Realizing that truth is the first step to moving past it and appreciating yourself as the beautiful human being you are.

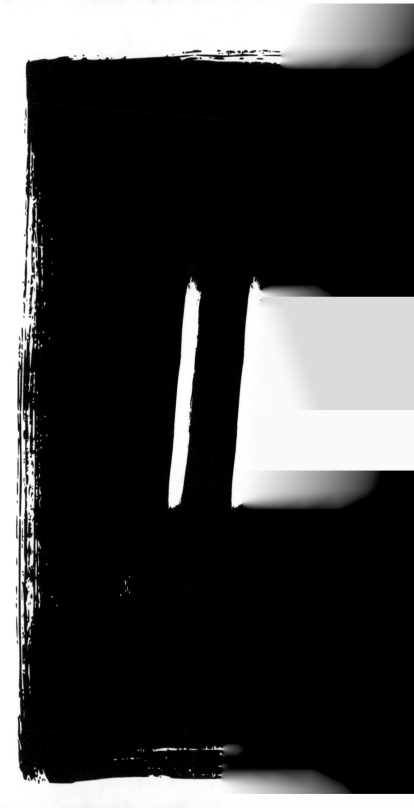

Can the Tide Be Turned?

Beauty is—and always has been—a central theme of human existence. We are all hardwired to look for beauty in a mate and potential co-creator of beautiful children; it's part of how a species evolves and continues. And there's nothing wrong with that!

Somewhere around the dawn of the advertising age, in the 18th century, the perception of beauty shifted from personal and cultural perceptions to more of a uniform standard pushed upon everyone by the fashion and cosmetics industries, and later by other industries including fitness, diet, and even the plastic surgery industry.

Now, some 300 years later, when it feels like the pressure to be beautiful is out of control thanks to the ubiquity of media, especially the metaverse, **there are positive signs of the tide slowly beginning to turn.**

Some celebrities, for whom appearing beautiful is understood to be part of the job, are starting to push back.

In late 2021, the hit 1990s television show *Sex and the City* rebooted with most of the original cast. The series centers around the lives of women who back in the 90s and early 2000s were in their early thirties. Obviously, they aged, and the co-stars received criticism for how their physical appearances changed.

In response, actress Sarah Jessica Parker said in a *Vogue* interview, "It almost feels as if people don't want us to be perfectly OK with where we are, as if they almost enjoy us being pained by who we are today, whether we choose to age naturally and not look perfect, or whether you do something if that makes you feel better."

"I know what I look like. I have no choice," she added. "What am I going to do about it? Stop aging? Disappear?"[1]

Grey's Anatomy star, Ellen Pompeo, shared similar sentiments on aging and beauty. "I think when you're in your 20s and 30s, you're super obsessed with your looks because you don't have any other wisdom...I have the wisdom to know that growing old is a privilege that not everyone is afforded. If my physical beauty is the only thing that leaves me, and my health and my family stay, then that is what's really important to me."[2]

It's not just aging beauty that is prompting the push-back. Jameela Jamil, a thirty-something actress of Pakistani descent, is outspoken about body positivity and transparency in social media. In one Instagram post, in which she shared an unfiltered photo of herself, she wrote, "I have stretch marks all over my body...they are a sign my body dared to take up extra space in a society that demands our eternal thinness. They are my badge of honor for resisting society's weaponizing of the female form."[3]

Ashley Graham is a *Sports Illustrated* swimsuit cover model at 5'9" and nearly 200 pounds. Does that surprise you? The magazine actually made history by putting her on its cover in 2016, another example of the slow movement our society is beginning to make away from the long-held traditional beauty standards. Ashley embraces her so-called plus-sized beauty and speaks out as a body-positive icon for women of all sizes. She shared a photo on Instagram capturing her stretch marks and cellulite and captioned, "I workout. I do my best to eat well. I love the skin I'm in. And I'm not ashamed of a few lumps, bumps, or cellulite…and you shouldn't be either."

Superstar singer Alicia Keys made the decision years into her career to no longer go glam. In an interview on *Today*, Keys said that choosing to opt-out of the makeup narrative is empowering:

The thing is... it kinda came from because we put so many limitations on ourselves, we put limitations on each other, society puts limitations on us, and in a lot of ways, I'm sick of it, I'm over it. And that's, in a lot of ways, what the music is about; it's about being our own unique selves, because we each have something that no one else has and it would be so amazing to embrace each other, how we are. I love makeup! I love my lip gloss, I love my blush, I love my eyeliner. It's not about that. But at the same time, I don't want to feel beholden...to have to do it. I just wanna be honest to myself, and all of us should be honest to ourselves. Just be yourself and have a great time, and do what makes you feel good as opposed to trying to please every damn body.[4]

Signs of Change

With more influencers beginning to push back on the traditional beauty standards, some companies have started to respond in positive ways. Around the same time *Sports Illustrated* began featuring plus-sized models, fashion lingerie retailer Aerie committed to no airbrushing "Aerie Real" advertising. The response was tremendously favorable, to the point of becoming a threat to the lingerie company probably best known for its airbrushed models—Victoria's Secret.[5]

"By December 2020, Victoria's Secret's market share had fallen to 19% in the U.S. women's intimate clothing space, compared to 32% in 2015. While it still has a higher share than any other brand, the company has undoubtedly fallen from grace."[6]

The Shiseido cosmetics company made some groundbreaking changes at that time, too, by overhauling its products, advertising, models, and even brand logo to align with their desire to make beauty "a positive force in the world." In a statement, the company advocated for an empathy "born when people recognize the diversity of beauty, respect the beauty present in one another, and realize the infinite nature of beauty."[7]

Glow Recipe, a Korean-American skincare brand that popularized the concept of *glass skin* among Western consumers, now avoids terms like flawless, poreless, ageless, anti-wrinkle, anti-aging, and perfect across all brand touchpoints. "It goes back to our values as a brand, which is being grounded in inclusion and making sure that every one of our customers feels reflected in our marketing, where we've never retouched our images and also ask the influencers we work with not to either," says co-founder Christine Chang.[8]

One of the biggest companies to get on board with making positive changes in the concept of beauty is Unilever, parent company to Dove. Their company Beauty Vision Statement declares, "Through our beauty and personal care brands, we're taking action to drive positive change. We're setting out to transform the systems that hold individuals back—by advocating new policies, laws, and social norms that will promote inclusion, health, and wellbeing for all members of society."[9]

Their actions back up their vision. Almost everyone is familiar with the widespread Dove Real Beauty campaigns which launched back in 2004 and continue to this day. The goal of every campaign is to "make women feel comfortable in the skin they are in and to create a world where beauty is a source of confidence and not anxiety."[10]

Given that one of the biggest sources of negative beauty messaging today is social media, Dove targeted one particular campaign, #speakbeautiful, at Twitter users. The goal of the campaign was to encourage women to realize the role our online words play in impacting our confidence and self-esteem.

Their research showed that in one year alone, **over five million negative body image tweets were posted**, yet only 9% of women said they posted negative comments. They uncovered the fact that women were not realizing their messages and posts were contributing to negative mindsets and behavior about beauty.[11]

With the #speakbeautiful campaign, Dove and Twitter leveraged technology that identified negative comments about beauty and body image, and then Dove would send non-automated responses which included advice and encouragement to be more positive and speak with more confidence, optimism, and kindness about beauty. The campaign ignited a positive conversation about body image and showcased Dove's work as a champion of positive body image for women.

Getting real about beauty turned Italian beautician Cristina Fogazzi's internet startup into a very wealthy beauty brand worth nearly $60 million—and she hasn't even begun to expand outside of her country yet! She got her start writing a no-nonsense, lighthearted beauty advice blog called *The Cynical Beautician*. Her messaging resonated with the women she reached: "I have a belly, but it is not contagious, and if you have supermodel legs, don't follow me."

As a result of her refreshing honesty when it comes to real beauty, women are lining up—literally—to buy her products, which she very openly claims are not magical:

One day, I had the opportunity to get a corner in the Rinascente department store in Milan. The morning of the opening, my staff and I arrived nice and early, only to find a big queue of women outside. When they saw me and started shouting 'Cinica!' I realized that they were there for us... There is no cream able to make stretch marks disappear. Same thing for wrinkles, I am afraid. Creams can minimize them, make your skin better-looking. But believe me, whoever promises otherwise is talking nonsense.[2]

Embrace Your True Beauty

It is encouraging to see some celebrities and businesses begin to slowly influence the positive trend toward accepting that true beauty does not necessarily align with the artificial beauty standards which have permeated cultures around the world for centuries. But it's going to take the power of every-day people to keep pushing that pendulum in the right direction. And that includes you.

It starts with embracing your own beauty. I hope you have taken to heart what I've shared in earlier chapters and feel empowered to choose the voices that influence you and see yourself as you really are—beautiful.

When you recognize your own beauty, you are better able to share the positive messaging with others. I make a point of genuinely complimenting some-thing about the beauty of every person who comes into my office for a consultation—and often people I just meet while I'm out and about! You can always find something beautiful to compliment:

Your haircut is amazing!
You have the prettiest eyes!
That outfit looks fantastic on you!

The awesome side effect of complimenting someone is how great it makes you feel when you see them smile! So while you're spreading beauty positivity, **you're feeling even better about yourself.**

And I'm not a plastic surgeon saying you have to get plastic surgery to feel better about yourself. I'm also not saying *not* to get plastic surgery. I'm saying life is about the energy we put into it.

I have seen people undergo a subtle Scarless Nose™ rhinoplasty with me and watched it transform their life—like a flower blooming. They finally believe more in themselves and exude the confidence that was always there hiding under the insecurity of the bump on their nose. I watch these patients chase their dreams, practice gratitude, and live unleashed lives after these transformations.

But I also see patients who undergo the same procedure and nothing changes. Sometimes it makes them even less confident and more hyper-focused on their flaws. It sometimes leads them down a dangerous spiral of negative thoughts and hyper-focus on micro-millimeter flaws with their surgical results or with other new issues.

The difference between these patients isn't their surgical results; **it's their mindset** before the procedure even happens. Where we focus our energy will eventually create a similar outcome. Positive energy towards oneself usually generates positive outcomes for one's life. Similarly, negative energy towards oneself usually generates negative outcomes.

In today's world, we tend to focus on the outcome instead of the process. We focus on achieving goals and being finished. We want happiness or beauty as an end goal to be achieved so we can put the trophy on our mantle and look at it with pride.

Unfortunately, that is not how life works. Ask any former Olympic gold medalist—the happiness of the medal fades with time because the pursuit was where the real passion and purpose always lived. Happiness, like feeling beautiful, is a moving target that you never win or achieve. The true measure of feeling happy or feeling beautiful is striving to achieve it daily, with a positive purpose.

Happiness, like feeling beautiful, is a moving target that you never win or achieve. The true measure of feeling happy or feeling beautiful is striving to achieve it daily, with a positive purpose.

Output is greater than Outcome. How much *effort and energy* is spent toward the positive focus is really all that matters. The outcome generated from it is totally out of our control. And that which we can't control, we must learn to let go of emotionally. So we must remember to not focus so much on how we *look*, but instead, put in the work every day toward how we *feel*, because that is where our control truly lies.

It's also important to remember that **everyone struggles with feeling beautiful some days**. When that moment of feeling ugly strikes, it's a lonely moment and sometimes alienates us from our peers as we feel self-conscious, which makes us naturally draw away.

Ironically, that moment is exactly what unifies us as humans—the universal struggle to want to feel more beautiful, to feel more confident, to feel happier. It affects people in different ways. Some only feel that self-conscious "less than" feeling when they want to wear their favorite suit and it feels tighter than when they bought it. Some feel it every day when they look in the mirror or when photos are being taken, and the anxiety of what they look like kicks in.

But in different ways, we all struggle with it, and instead of letting this feeling separate us, **it should be what makes us feel more connected and more human**. Knowing how universal the struggle is, we should all aim to be kinder and lift each other up instead of being part of the systemic problem that tears so many of us down.

In the end, I think all of us can appreciate a lesson about beauty that comes from people who are unable to observe physical beauty. In a viral YouTube video entitled "Blind People Describe Beauty", four blind people are interviewed about their concept of beauty. While they admit that they aren't immune to some of the more common desires around beauty—appreciating when someone tells them they look good, etc.— they also embrace the intangibles:

"I guess other senses kick in...just the tenderness, the smoothness...it's the little things. It's like a sound, or a scent, or a touch...and it all builds into this generalized thing. I don't look at it as visual beauty. I receive it as what they project to me, their heart. I don't think vision really plays that big of a role in beauty."[13]

Think about that for a moment. **If you couldn't see your imperfections, how would you feel?** Better or Worse? Maybe it's up to us that what we visualize and focus on every day controls how we feel. Focusing on our insecurities will always make us feel weaker. Instead, if we consciously chose to focus on our strengths, our sources of confidence, and practice gratitude routinely, we would be able to lift ourselves into a higher state of positivity and do the same for all those around us.

Because in the end, it's not about *looking* beautiful, it's about *feeling* beautiful. And everyone can and should feel beautiful—because you truly are.

Beauty Notes

* In our present day and age,
  when it feels like the pressure
  to be beautiful is out of control
  thanks to the ubiquity of media,
  especially the metaverse, there
  are positive signs of the tide
  slowly beginning to turn.

* Some models, actors, and social
  media influencers are beginning
  to push back on the traditional
  beauty standards, and a few
  companies have also begun
  to respond in positive ways.

* When you recognize your own
  beauty, you are better able to
  share the positive messaging
  with others. You can always find
  something beautiful to compliment:

- Your haircut is amazing!
- You have the prettiest eyes!
- That outfit looks fantastic on you!

The awesome side effect of complimenting someone is how great it makes you feel when you see them smile! So while you're spreading beauty positivity, you're feeling even better about yourself.

* In different ways, we all struggle with feeling less than beautiful sometimes, and instead of letting this feeling separate us, it should be what makes us feel more connected and more human. Knowing how universal the struggle is, we should all aim to be kinder and lift each other up instead of being part of the systemic problem that tears so many of us down.

Acknowledgments

I would like to thank my patients who have opened their hearts to me, with their deepest insecurities, often shared with no one else. Their pure conversations allowed me to better understand the human psyche in terms of concepts of beauty. Through this book, I am able to share these invaluable lessons for the world to benefit from. I would like to thank my wife, Puja, and my daughter, Maya, for giving me the deepest purpose my life has ever had. I also thank my amazing mentors including Dr. Raj Kanodia for teaching me the wisest life lessons beyond the world of plastic surgery. I thank my parents for raising me with awareness, purpose, and ethical values every day.

About the Author

Deepak Dugar, MD is a Beverly Hills Celebrity Plastic Surgeon who isn't afraid to say no to his patients. He has become globally known for his expertise in Scarless Nose™ rhinoplasty. But more often than not, Dr. Dugar's real talent lies in his ability to discern which patients need a procedure, and which simply need to talk.

After more than 10,000 consultations with patients from around the world, Dr. Dugar knows the conversation can often be more profound and powerful than any surgical outcome. Dr. Dugar wants to initiate that conversation with you by bringing awareness to how beautiful you already are, even if traditional beauty standards have you believing otherwise.

In addition to being published in internationally acclaimed peer-reviewed journals and lecturing at national medical conferences around the country,

Dr. Dugar has served as a Medical Contributor and Advisor to The Doctors, E! News, Sirius XM Radio, Huffington Post, Allure Magazine, and others who look to him for expertise in beauty.

Dr. Dugar is married to his college sweetheart, Dr. Puja Roy, who performs Anesthesiology at the Beverly Hills Rhinoplasty Center™. During their free time, Drs. Dugar and Roy enjoy spending time with their family, the outdoor lifestyle of Los Angeles, and traveling the world.

Notes

Chapter 1

1. Crawford, Cindy, and Katherine O'Leary. *Becoming*. Rizzoli, 2015, 25.

2. Crawford, *Becoming*, 316.

Chapter 2

1. Katharine Phillips, "Prevalence of BDD", accessed February, 18, 2022, https://bdd.iocdf.org/professionals/prevalence/#:~:text=Body%20 Dysmorphic%20Disorder%20affects%201.7,about%201%20in%20 50%20people.

2. Lifespan. "Does cosmetic surgery help body dysmorphic disorder?." ScienceDaily., accessed February 16, 2022, www.sciencedaily.com/ releases/2010/08/100811101424.htm.

3. Minda Zetlin. "Want Your Daughters to Grow Up Successful and Happy? Help Them Stop Doing This 1 Thing." February 20, 2017, https://www.inc.com/minda-zetlin/want-to-raise-high-achieving-daughters-help-them-stop-doing-this.html.

4. "Body Image: List of Fact, Figures, and Statistics", Beauty School Directory, accessed February 18, 2022, https://www. beautyschoolsdirectory.com/blog/body-image-statistics.

5. "Our Research", Dove, accessed February 18, 2022, https://www.dove. com/us/en/stories/about-dove/our-research.html.

6. Kelly Braun, "Jennifer Aniston Admits She's 'Never Thought' Of Herself As 'Glamorous'", December 28, 2018, https://www. closerweekly.com/posts/jennifer-aniston-admits-shes-never-thought-of-herself-as-glamorous/ .

7. "Jennifer Lopez talks body image and overcoming her insecurities", HELLOMAGAZINE.COM, lJune 20, 2016, https://www.hellomagazine. com/healthandbeauty/health-and-fitness/2016062031994/ jennifer-lopez-talks-overcoming-insecurities-and-embracing-her-body/.

8. Kelcie Willis, "Beyonce talks body image, relationships, representation in Vogue September issue", August 6, 2018, https://www.ajc.com/entertainment/beyonce-talks-body-image-relationships-representation-vogue-september-issue/zhLoCSTTL8oRRlosPHJXnI/.

9. Christopher Rosa, "Male Celebrities Who Opened Up About Their Body Image Issues", March 24, 2016, http://www.vh1.com/news/253155/male-celebrities-body-image/.

10. Christopher Rosa, "Male Celebrities Who Opened Up About Their Body Image Issues"

11. The nerve blog, "The Brain's Perception of Beauty", 11, 2017, https://sites.bu.edu/ombs/2017/10/11/the-brains-perception-of-beauty/.

12. Aditya Shukla, "Global highlights from research on attractiveness, aesthetic perception, and ugliness (TL;DR)", April 10, 2021, https://cognitiontoday.com/beautiful-science-of-ugliness-reveals-uncomfortable-truths-about-ugly-beauty-biases/#Global_highlights_from_research_on_attractiveness_aesthetic_perception_and_ugliness_TLDR.

Chapter 3

1. "Himba Women - the Most Beautiful Tribe of Africa", Beauty Around, Accessed February 21, 2022, http://beauty-around.com/en/drugie-reitingi/item/1788-beautiful-himba-woman#comments.

2. "Himba People", Wikipedia, last modified February 13, 2022, https://en.wikipedia.org/wiki/Himba_people.

Chapter 4

1. Yosh Jefferson, "Facial beauty--establishing a universal standard.", accessed February 18, 2022, https://pubmed.ncbi.nlm.nih.gov/15085778/.

2. Allison Pearce Stevens, "What makes a pretty face?", December 2, 2016, https://www.sciencenewsforstudents.org/article/what-makes-pretty-face.

3. Tbd

4. "Cosmetics", AdAge, September 15, 2003, https://adage.com/article/adage-encyclopedia/cosmetics/98602.

5. "Cosmetics", AdAge.

6. "Body Image Survey Results", House of Commons, September 23, 2020, https://committees.parliament.uk/publications/2691/documents/26657/d.

7. Daniel B. Yarosh, "Perception and Deception: Human Beauty and the Brain", April 9. 2019, https://www.ncbi.nlm.nih.gov/pmc/articles/PMC6523404/.

Chapter 5

1. Julie Zeilinger, "The Disturbing Effect Our Beauty Standards Have on Women Across the World", February 27, 2015, https://www.mic.com/articles/111228/how-western-beauty-ideals-are-hurting-women-across-the-globe.

2. "Western Beauty Pressures and Their Impact on Young University Women", International Journal of Gender and Women's Studies, December 2018, http://ijgws.com/journals/ijgws/Vol_6_No_2_December_2018/1.pdf.

3. Nancy Matsumoto, "How the Asian Pop Culture Boom Is Feeding Eating Disorders", September 16, 2014, https://www.psychologytoday.com/us/blog/eating-disorders-news/201409/how-the-asian-pop-culture-boom-is-feeding-eating-disorders.

4. Sandy Kobrin, "Restoring Virginity Becomes Risky Business", May 22, 2005, https://womensenews.org/2005/05/restoring-virginity-becomes-risky-business/.

5. Mohamad Kashmar, "Consensus Opinions on Facial Beauty and Implications for Aesthetic Treatment in Middle Eastern Women", last modified April 7, 2019, https://www.ncbi.nlm.nih.gov/pmc/articles/PMC6554175/.

6. Parisa Hashempour, "Middle Easter looks are 'trending', but where does that leave Middle Eastern women?", November 22, 2020, https://gal-dem.com/middle-eastern-beauty-trend/.

7. Amanda Mitchell, "Why Brazilian Lymphatic Drainage Massages Have Become a Celebrity Fave", last modified January 11, 2022, https://www.byrdie.com/brazilian-lymphatic-drainage-massage-5101241.

8. Paulo Gomes, "Brazil Registers More Than 180 Rapes per Day, The Highest since 2019", September 11, 2019, https://www1.folha.uol.com.br/internacional/en/brazil/2019/09/brazil-registers-more-than-180-rapes-per-day-the-highest-since-2009.shtml#:~:text=Brazil%20registered%20more%20than%2066%2C000,in%20the%20Brazilian%20Penal%20Code.

9. "Girls Challenge Rape Culture in Brazil", Plan International, accessed February 18, 2022, https://plan-international.org/advancing-global-goals-girls-brazil.

10. Khesraw Majidi, "Norms of Beauty in India Fair is Beautiful: A Legacy of Colonialism and Globalization", June 22, 2020, http://thelionandthehunter.org/norms-of-beauty-in-india-fair-is-beautiful-a-legacy-of-colonialism-and-globalization/#:~:text=As%20the%20ideal%20Indian%20woman,last%20in%20India%20for%20centuries.

11. Tony Joseph, "New reports clearly confirm 'Arya' migrations into India", last modified September 14, 2019, https://www.thehindu.com/society/history-and-culture/theres-no-confusion-the-new-reports-clearly-confirm-arya-migration-into-india/article29409611.ece.

12. Anuja Premika, "India and its UN-FAIR Beauty Standards | Documentary", November 6, 2019, https://www.youtube.com/watch?v=k47Hj994xN4.

13. Anuja Premika, "India and its UN-FAIR Beauty Standards | Documentary"

14. "India's multibillion-dollar skin lightening industry under fire as Indians seek whiter shade of pale", April 27, 2017, https://ww.fashionnetwork.com/news/India-s-multibillion-dollar-skin-lightening-industry-under-fire-as-indians-seek-whiter-shade-of-pale,821354.html.

15. Anuja Premika, "India and its UN-FAIR Beauty Standards | Documentary"

16. Julie Zeilinger, "The Disturbing Effect Our Beauty Standards Have on Women Across the World"

17. Julie Zeilinger, "The Disturbing Effect Our Beauty Standards Have on Women Across the World"

18. Hazel Lutz, "India: Clothing and Adornment", date accessed February 18, 2022, https://fashion-history.lovetoknow.com/clothing-around-world/india-clothing-adornment.

19. Varsha Patel, "For Indian Women, The Pressure To Look Perfect Is A Problem Born At Home", September 20, 2019, https://www.refinery29.com/en-gb/indian-asian-beauty-standrards-pressure.

20. "The Countries With The Largest Number Of Cosmetic Surgeries", Cosmetic Surgery Solicitors, October 7, 2020, https://www.cosmeticsurgerysolicitors.co.uk/news/countries-largest-number-cosmetic-surgeries.

21. Diana-Abasi Ibanga, "The Concept of Beauty in African Philosophy", September 2017, https://www.jpanafrican.org/docs/vol10no7/10.7-16-Ibanga-final.pdf.

22. Noam Schulman, "Beauty Standards From The Most Remote Locations", October 31, 2019, https://magazine.calcalistech.com/culture/1429511904/beauty-standards-from-the-most-remote-locations/?org=true&utm_source=facebook&utm_campaign=zx-ww-shareclt-orgcsposhareclt1m.

23. "More than half of sub-Saharan Africans lack access to electricity", The Economist, November 13, 2019, https://www.economist.com/graphic-detail/2019/11/13/more-than-half-of-sub-saharan-africans-lack-access-to-electricity.

Chapter 6

1. Ron Marshall, "How Many Ads Do We See In One Day?", September 10, 2015, https://www.redcrowmarketing.com/2015/09/10/many-ads-see-one-day/.

2. Kilbourne, Jean, Can't Buy My Love: How Advertising Changes the Way We Think and Feel. New York: Simon & Schuster, 2000.

3. "How do beauty product ads affect consumer self esteem and purchasing?", University of Chicago Press Journals, October 26, 2010, https://www.sciencedaily.com/releases/2010/10/101018163112.htm.

4. Sam Escobar, "The Number of Makeup Products the Average Woman Owns Is Just Plain Shocking", October 14, 2015, https://www.goodhousekeeping.com/beauty/makeup/a34976/average-makeup-products-owned/.

5. Charles Sternberg, "Global Cosmetics Industry Forecasted to Reach $463.5 Billion by 2027", March 15, 2021, https://www.beautypackaging.com/contents/view_breaking-news/2021-03-15/global-cosmetics-industry-forecasted-to-reach-4635-billion-by-2027/#:~:text=According%20to%20a%20recent%20report,5.3%25%20from%202021%20to%202027.

6. "Beauty Advertising - Message and Content", Stockholm School of Economics, accessed 18, 2022, http://arc.hhs.se/download.aspx?mediumid=1685.

7. Jacquelyn Schlabach, "Chanel Fiscal Year 2020 Results", June 15, 2021, https://www.gcimagazine.com/brands-products/news/news/21862126/chanel-fiscal-year-2020-results.

8. Mark Sweney, "L'Oréal's Julia Roberts and Christy Turlington ad campaigns banned", July 26, 2011, https://www.theguardian.com/media/2011/jul/27/loreal-julia-roberts-ad-banned.

9. Mark Sweney, "L'Oréal's Julia Roberts and Christy Turlington ad campaigns banned"

10. "Don't Fall for False Advertisement When it Comes to Fashion", Professor's House, accessed February 18, 2022, https://www.professorshouse.com/dont-fall-for-false-advertisement-when-it-comes-to-fashion/.

11. "The Business of Fashion: 7 Surprising Facts About The Fashion Industry", Social Media Sun, accessed February 18, 2022, https://socialmediasun.com/the-business-of-fashion-7-surprising-facts-about-the-fashion-industry/.

12. Gabby Neal, "5 FALSE ADVERTISING TRICKS STILL USED IN THE INDUSTRY", accessed February 18, 2022, https://www.allmyfriendsaremodels.com/false-advertising-fashion/.

13. "Don't Fall for False Advertisement When it Comes to Fashion", Professor's House

14. John Holmes, "Losing 25,000 to Hunger Everyday", accessed February 18, 2022, https://www.un.org/en/chronicle/article/losing-25000-hunger-every-day#:~:text=Each%20day%2C%2025%2C000%20people%2C%20including,million%20into%20poverty%20and%20hunger.

15. "The $72 Billion Weight Loss & Diet Control Market in the United States, 2019-2023 - Why Meal Replacements are Still Booming, but Not OTC Diet Pills - ResearchAndMarkets.com", Business Wire, February 25, 2019, https://www.businesswire.com/news/home/20190225005455/en/The-72-Billion-Weight-Loss-Diet-Control-Market-in-the-United-States-2019-2023---Why-Meal-Replacements-are-Still-Booming-but-Not-OTC-Diet-Pills---ResearchAndMarkets.com.

16. "Weight Loss Marketer TV Spend in 2016 Hits $100M", iSpot.tv, March 10, 2016, https://www.nexttv.com/news/weight-loss-marketer-tv-spend-2016-hits-100m-154541.

17. Danna Ethan, "An analysis of weight loss articles and advertisements in mainstream women's health and fitness magazines", June 11, 2016, https://www.ncbi.nlm.nih.gov/pmc/articles/PMC4932226/.

18. "The Truth Behind Weight Loss Ads", Federal Trade Commission, accessed February 18, 2022, https://www.consumer.ftc.gov/articles/truth-behind-weight-loss-ads-0.

19. Savannah Greenfield, "When Beauty is the Beast: The Effects of Beauty Propaganda on Female Consumers", August 2018, https://digitalcommons.unomaha.edu/cgi/viewcontent.cgi?article=1028&context=university_honors_program.

20. "Cosmetic Surgery and Procedure Market Worth $43.9 Billion by 2025" Grand View Research, accessed February 18, 2022, https://www.grandviewresearch.com/press-release/global-cosmetic-surgery-procedure-market.

21. Lori Bahnmueller, "Cosmetic Surgery Advertising: The changing face of medical marketing", September 13, 2018, https://brogan.com/blog/cosmetic-surgery-advertising-changing-face-medical-marketing/.

22. Lori Bahnmueller, "Cosmetic Surgery Advertising: The changing face of medical marketing"

23. Dina Gerdeman, "Lipstick Tips: How Influencers Are Making Over Beauty Marketing", August 26, 2019, https://hbswk.hbs.edu/item/lipstick-tips-how-influencers-are-making-over-beauty-marketing.

24. Ibid

25. Ibid

26. Ibid

27. Rose Lagace, "The Devil Wears Prada Cerulean Sweater Monolog", July 17, 2017, https://artdepartmental.com/blog/devil-wears-prada-cerulean-monologue/.

Chapter 1

1. "Social Media Fact Sheet", Pew Research Center, April 7, 2021, https://www.pewresearch.org/internet/fact-sheet/social-media/?menuItem=b14b718d-7ab6-46f4-b447-0abd510f4180.

2. Kara Cutruzulla, "Here's Why You Can't Stop Scrolling on Your Phone", June 20 2019, https://advice.theshineapp.com/articles/heres-why-you-cant-stop-scrolling-on-your-phone/.

3. Salome Phelamei, "What happens to your body when you look at your phone first thing in the morning?", November 7, 2019, https://www.timesnownews.com/health/article/what-happens-to-your-body-when-you-look-at-your-phone-first-thing-in-the-morning/512627#:~:text=According%20to%20a%20research%20study,health%20and%20productivity%20as%20well.

4. "Branwell Moffat Director of CX Consulting KPS Digital", The Future of Customer Engagement and Experience, accessed February 18, 2022, https://www.the-future-of-commerce.com/contributor/branwell-moffat/.

5. Ntainu Obiora, "The dark side of social media: How unrealistic beauty standards are causing identity issues.", November 28, 2021, https://www.pulse.ng/lifestyle/beauty-health/the-dark-side-of-social-media-how-unrealistic-beauty-standards-are-causing-identity/hv4tffb.

6. Mavis Henriques and Debasis Patnaik, "Social Media and Its Effect on Beauty", September 21, 2020, https://www.intechopen.com/chapters/73271.

7. Jeremy Gray, "Norway passes law requiring influences to label retouched photos on social media", July 9, 2021, https://www.dpreview.com/news/1157704583/norway-passes-law-requiring-influencers-to-label-retouched-photos-on-social-media.

8. Nalina Eggert, "Is she Photoshopped? In France, they now have to tell you", September 30, 2017, https://www.bbc.com/news/world-europe-41443027.

9. Aaron Horwath, "Photoshop, Models, and the Law: How Far is Too Far?", accessed February 18, 2022, https://www.pixelz.com/blog/photoshop-models-laws/.

Chapter 8

1. Heather Corinna, "Why Do We Go to Such Lengths to Look Young", June 1, 2021, https://www.damemagazine.com/2021/06/01/why-do-we-go-to-such-lengths-to-look-young/.

2. "ANTI-AGING MARKET - GROWTH, TRENDS, COVID-19 IMPACT, AND FORECASTS (2022 - 2027)", Modor Intelligence, accessed February 18, 2022, https://www.mordorintelligence.com/industry-reports/anti-aging-market.

3. Heather Corinna, "Why Do We Go to Such Lengths to Look Young"

4. Sabrina Felson, MD, "14 Things No One Tells You About Aging", June 12, 2020, https://www.webmd.com/healthy-aging/ss/slideshow-aging-surprises.

5. Sabrina Felson, MD, "14 Things No One Tells You About Aging"

6. Eustacia Huen, "World's Most Expensive Anti-Aging Serum Costs $1,800 Per Ounce", January 31, 2017, https://www.forbes.com/sites/eustaciahuen/2017/01/31/worlds-most-expensive-anti-aging-serum-costs-1800-per-ounce/?sh=4e873661bc5c.

7. Eustacia Huen, "World's Most Expensive Anti-Aging Serum Costs $1,800 Per Ounce"

8. Eustacia Huen, "World's Most Expensive Anti-Aging Serum Costs $1,800 Per Ounce"

9. "L'Oréal Settles FTC Charges Alleging Deceptive Advertising for Anti-Aging Cosmetics", Federal Trade Comission, June 30 2014, https://www.ftc.gov/news-events/press-releases/2014/06/loreal-settles-ftc-charges-alleging-deceptive-advertising-anti.

10. Gabriella Ulloa, "Are There Benefits to Collagen Supplements", November 9, 2019, https://www.nytimes.com/2019/11/09/style/self-care/collagen-benefits.html.

11. Danielle Friedman, "Men's Hair Loss is a Multi-Billion Dollar Industry (and Growing)", October 2, 2019, https://www.instyle.com/hair/mens-hair-loss-industry-balding.

12. NU SKIN INTERNATIONAL, INC., ET AL., Federal Trace Comission, accessed February 18, 2022, https://www.ftc.gov/sites/default/files/documents/commission_decision_volumes/volume-117/ftc_volume_decision_117_january_-_june_1994pages_316_-_418.pdf.

Chapter 9

1. Alice Walker, *Beauty"When the Other Dancer Is the Self.* Accessed Feb 21, 2022, https://www.oleanschools.org/cms/lib/NY19000263/Centricity/Domain/166/Beauty.pdf

2. Kristin Salaky, "11 scientific ways to make yourself look and feel more attractive", August 9, 2017, https://www.insider.com/ways-to-look-feel-more-attractive-confident-2017-8.

3. Catherine Moore, "Positive Daily Affirmations: Is There Science Behind It?", February 14, 2022, https://positivepsychology.com/daily-affirmations/.

4. Kristin Salaky, "11 scientific ways to make yourself look and feel more attractive"

5. Kristin Salaky, "11 scientific ways to make yourself look and feel more attractive"

6. Dana R. Carney, Amy J.C. Cuddy, Andy J. Yap, Power Posing: Brief Nonverbal Displays Affect Neuroendocrine Levels and Risk Tolerance, September 20, 2010, https://journals.sagepub.com/doi/abs/10.1177/0956797610383437?journalCode=pssa.

7. Oprah Winfrey, Cybill Shepherd Comes Clean About Aging, accessed February 18, 2022, https://www.oprah.com/oprahs-lifeclass/cybill-shepherd-comes-clean-about-aging-video.

8. Alice Hart-Davis, "Yes, any woman can look better at 50 than 20 and I'm proof!: Alice Hart-Davis shares the secrets to a youthful appearance", October 15, 2017, https://www.dailymail.co.uk/femail/article-4982972/Any-woman-look-better-50-20-m-proof.html.

Chapter 10

1. "What Makes "The Ugliest Woman in the World" Feel Beautiful | Dispelling Beauty Myths | Allure", Allure, October 19, 2016, https://www.youtube.com/watch?v=ztJkD7-Vtks.

2. Lizzie Velasquez, "How Do YOU Define Yourself Lizzie Velasquez at TEDxAustinWomen", December 20, 2013, https://www.youtube.com/watch?v=c62Aqdlzvqk.

3. Lizzie Velasquez, "How Do YOU Define Yourself Lizzie Velasquez at TEDxAustinWomen"

4. "What Makes "The Ugliest Woman in the World" Feel Beautiful | Dispelling Beauty Myths | Allure", Allure

5. "Lillie Velasquez on Hitting Rock Bottom and the Pressure to Be a "Superhero" | Pretty Unfiltered", Popsugar, August 2, 2017, https://www.youtube.com/watch?v=91_4IBpUpb8.

6. Nichole Wood-Barcalow, Tracy Tylka andCasey Judge, *Positive Body Image Workbook* (Cambridge University Press, 2021), Chapter 17.

7. Nichole Wood-Barcalow, Tracy Tylka andCasey Judge, *Positive Body Image Workbook* (Cambridge University Press, 2021), Chapter 17.

8. "Mom Stop Trashing My Appearance - It's Bad for the Grandkids", Parentcc November 3, 2016, https://www.parent.com/blogs/conversations/mom-stop-trashing-my-appearance-its-bad-for-the-grandkids.

9. "Mom Stop Trashing My Appearance - It's Bad for the Grandkids", Parentcc

10. Ornella Evans, Sarah E. Stutterheim, Jessica M. Alleva, "Protective filtering: A qualitative study on the cognitive strategies young women use to promote positive body image in the face of beauty-ideal imagery on Instagram", Decemb 2021, https://www.sciencedirect.com/science/article/pii/S1740144521000917.

11. Amber Karnes, "Yoga Turned My Body Into A Place I Could Call Home", accessed February 18, 2022, https://yogainternational.com/article/view/body-acceptance-through-yoga.

Chapter 11

1. Lauren Cox, "Sarah Jessica Parker slams 'misogynist' comments about aging looks", November 7, 2021, https://pagesix.com/2021/11/07/sarah-jessica-parker-slams-misogynist-comments-about-ageism/.

2. Sophie Dodd, "'You Are More Than a Number on a Scale': Stars Who Are Redefining How We Talk About Beauty", April 22, 2019, https://news.yahoo.com/more-number-scale-stars-redefining-184252243.html?guccounter=1&guce_referrer=aHR0cHM6Ly93d3cuZ29vZ2xlLmNvbS88&guce_referrer_sig=AQAAAB xsazUY3YmPtBQjmTLfIILh3F50Ygo6xrCY-Cb5-46CTrzAAvDRs6sdE4kmjISVW bh3fs1dCaLRxePGivXHlmLVJY6gxLjybxm-dFVgbx9DAyLScRNcxAbw9ei2gn2-FeWMHpu997_nUihfgoCIfLE4MyKXzZGcHNFvmyKWKaj2.

3. "21 Times Celebrities Challenged Beauty Standards by Sharing Their So-Called Flaws", Glamour, February 18, 2020, https://www.glamour.com/story/celebrities-whove-showed-us-th.

4. "Alicia Keys lights up TODAY with hits, 'empowering' take on beauty", The Today Show, January 17, 2020, https://www.today.com/popculture/alicia-keys-lights-today-hits-empowering-take-beauty-t102494

5. Krista Burton, "Victoria's Secret, your airbrushed grip on the lingerie world is loosening", March 4, 2019, https://www.theguardian.com/commentisfree/2019/mar/04/victorias-secret-airbrushed-grip-lingerie.

6. Amina Asim and Li Lu, "Cast Study: How Aerie won Gen Z and Victoria's Secret Market Share", November 9, 2021, https://www.glossy.co/fashion/case-study-how-aerie-won-gen-z-and-victorias-secrets-market-share/.

7. "Shiseido to reinvent itself as a "positive force"", Cosmetics Business, October 14, 2015, https://www.cosmeticsbusiness.com/news/article_page/Shiseido_to_reinvent_itself_as_a_positive_force/112745.

8. Glow Recipe, "We're all for having conversations and bringing light to what REAL skin is.", Facebook Posts, August 9, 2021, https://www.facebook.com/glowrecipe/photos/a.354580351376154/2826398444194320/?type=3.

9. "Our Positive Beauty vision for people and planet", Unilever, accessed February 18, 2022, https://www.unilever.com/brands/beauty-personal-care/our-positive-beauty-strategy/.

10. "Dove Campaign for Real Beauty", Wikipedia, accessed February 18, 2022, https://en.wikipedia.org/wiki/Dove_Campaign_for_Real_Beauty.

11. "THE POWER IS IN OUR HANDS TO #SPEAKBEAUTIFUL AND CHANGE THE CONVERSATION IN SOCIAL MEDIA", Dove, February 19, 2015, https://www.multivu.com/players/English/7447351-dove-twitter-speak-beautiful/.

12. "VeraLab got its start selling online two years ago and became profitable. Now, it's moved to physical locations.", Digital Commerce 360, accessed February 18, 2022, https://www.digitalcommerce360.com/2021/06/30/challenging-beauty-standards-ignites-cosmetics-brand/.

13. "Blind People Describe Beauty | Blind People Describe | Cut", Cut, September 12, 2017, https://www.youtube.com/watch?v=JO7X9ZP0Ap8.